nutrition periodization for athletes

Taking Traditional Sports Nutrition to the Next Level

BOB SEEBOHAR, MS, RD, CSCS

Bull Publishing Company
P.O. Box 1377
Boulder, CO 80306
(800) 676-2855
www.bullpub.com
ISBN 978-1-933503-65-3

Distributed to the trade by:
Independent Publishers Group
814 North Franklin Street
Chicago, IL 60610

Publisher: James Bull
Project Manager: Emily Sewell
Cover Design: Lightbourne, Inc.
Interior Design and Composition: Publication Services, Inc.

Library of Congress Cataloging-in-Publication Data

Seebohar, Bob.
    Nutrition periodization for endurance athletes : taking traditional
sports nutrition to the next level / Bob Seebohar. — 2nd ed.
        p. cm.
    Includes bibliographical references and index.
    ISBN 978-1-933503-65-3
    1. Athletes—Nutrition. I. Title.

  TX361.A8S44 2011
  613.2'024796—dc22
                            2010037565

10 9 8 7 6 5 4 3 2 1

Dedication

I have grown and learned quite a bit as a sport dietitian, coach, and athlete since the first edition of this book was published. This second edition is dedicated to all of the athletes with whom I have worked who have helped me understand the ever-changing aspects of sports nutrition and the different implementation strategies based on the sport and gender of the athlete.

—Bob Seebohar

Contents

List of Tables/Figures

LIST OF FIGURES

Introduction

A New Way of Thinking about Nutrition

FROM PAST TO PRESENT

Seven years have passed since the first edition of this book was published in 2004, and, in that time, a few things have changed in the sports nutrition and athletic performance worlds. With this, I have improved the second edition substantially by broadening the depth of using the nutrition periodization concept to many different types of sports and athletes. The first edition served as a complement to other sports nutrition books, whereas this edition provides athletes with everything they need to understand the concept and, most important, implement it during daily training. Each chapter is enhanced based on the latest research and my real-life "in the trenches" work with athletes, ranging from youth to Olympians, in many sports, including strength and power, aesthetic, weight-class, team, technical, and endurance.

Examples of Strength and Power Sports

- Weight lifting
- Bobsled
- Track and field (field events)

Examples of Aesthetic and Weight-Class Sports

- Gymnastics
- Figure skating
- Wrestling
- Boxing
- Tae Kwon Do

Examples of Team and Technical Sports

- Soccer
- Basketball
- Football
- Golf
- Baseball
- Volleyball
- Hockey

Examples of Endurance Sports

- Triathlon
- Cycling
- Running
- Swimming
- Cross-country skiing
- Biathlon
- Rowing
- Track and field (distance events)

The concept of nutrition periodization described in this book is still the most cutting-edge principle within sports nutrition and physical performance and is being implemented in more and more sports with great success.

ABOUT THIS BOOK

I like to challenge conventional wisdom and ask "why" quite often. This is what makes me so successful in delivering nutrition information to athletes. My combination of knowledge about the science and what works in real life is what sets this book apart from others. References reflect the sports nutrition messaging that is presented throughout this book, but you will also find my real-life examples of how this is applied to you, the athlete. At the end of the day, nutrition must work for you. It must assist you in enhancing your health, supporting a strong immune system, and improving performance.

I encourage you to leave behind your preconceived notions of sports nutrition before reading further. An open mind and the ability to want to apply the principles presented throughout this book are your biggest allies as you strive to improve yourself as an athlete.

To get the most out of this book, relinquish your traditional belief that nutrition is only important a few days or a week prior to, during, and immediately after your competition. This "old school" method of sports nutrition is very narrow in focus and does not normally address the true needs of athletes who are training and competing on a consistent basis. The "new school" way to approach using nutrition as your ally is to discover the benefits that a year-round, periodized nutrition plan bring you. You have specific physiological goals associated with each training cycle, such as increasing endurance, speed, strength, and power and improving technique, tactics, and economy; thus, you should have specific nutrition goals as well. Depending on your sport, your nutrition goals may include losing or gaining weight, decreasing body fat and increasing lean muscle mass, reducing inflammation and free radical production, and improving blood lipids. Your nutrition plan should support your training, not the other way around.

Think about that for a moment. Your eating program should support your training so that you are able to train efficiently and effectively to enhance your health and improve your performance. To elicit positive physiological responses, your nutrition must support your body's energy needs as they change with the varying training volume and intensity stressors in your training program throughout the year. My mantra, "Eat to train, don't train to eat,"™ becomes your guiding light.

Approach your training sessions with adequate fuel and hydration stores, and you will see physical benefits. There may be times, however, when you are not concerned with pre-hydrating before training, or when you are trying to improve your metabolic efficiency and therefore not eating during a training session, or when you do not follow the research-supported post-workout nutrition principles because your training cycle simply doesn't warrant it. This is the most important message throughout this book. Look at your nutrition as a function of your energy expenditure and physical goals associated with each training cycle to guide your nutritional choices.

Before you explore each chapter of this book, make sure that you are comfortable with the message in the previous paragraph. I cannot emphasize enough that you need to be able to think in the "new school" way about nutrition and your yearly training program. This may be a radical departure for you, and you may need to re-read chapters in order to leave your "old school" application of sports nutrition behind, but, in the end, it is worth it. Hundreds of athletes have proven this to me over the years and continue to do so. Why did it work so well for them? Because they were ready to accept new methods of using nutrition to support their training and take their performance to the next level.

PLAY BY PLAY

This book presents concepts and ideas that you may not have read about in other sports nutrition books. Chapter 1 provides an in-depth discussion of physical periodization so that you have a better idea of the history and, more important, the different methods that are used by coaches for athletes and teams. Knowing this information is the crucial first step in applying nutrition because there isn't just one physical periodization model, and thus, the nutrition plan is ever changing throughout a competition year based on the training stressors and goals.

Chapter 2 is probably the closest that this book gets to other sports nutrition books—by providing the background of the nutrients needed to sustain life. Having this foundational knowledge is crucial before applying nutrition periodization to sport.

Chapter 3 is the bread and butter of the book. You learn about the concept of nutrition periodization, and, more important, how to apply it to different athletes in different sports with different physical periodization models. This chapter is where I bring the nutrition periodization concept to life!

Chapter 4, "Body Weight and Performance," includes my in-depth approach to changing body weight and lean and fat mass in athletes. My approach is very different than that of any other sport dietitian, which will likely be a breath of fresh air for you. I present three different methods that you can use depending on your behavioral and personality styles and readiness to make a change. The information in this chapter will make you approach food differently by improving your awareness of the reasons behind why you eat rather than just going through the motions of using food as fuel.

Chapter 5 gives a behind-the-scenes account of the supplement industry and provides you with the information that you need to make better choices when selecting supplements. I also describe the three categories of supplements and which ones fit into each category so that you have a better understanding of how to navigate the very confusing world of supplements.

Chapter 6 includes some very important topics that all athletes need to consider at some point in their athletic lives. Many topics that often get lost in the educational messaging, such as inflammation, iron deficiency, and vegetarianism, are highlighted, with information on how to best use each principle to support your health and performance goals.

My approach to sports nutrition with athletes begins as a coach, athlete, and exercise physiologist. I understand sport from both the coaching and athletic side, and this knowledge helps me bring my sports nutrition expertise to athletes in a matter-of-fact method that produces results. Science guides the work I do with athletes, but being an athlete and a coach allows me to apply the science in real-life sport applications.

I wish you the best as you embark on your nutrition periodization journey and guarantee that, if you apply the principles you discover throughout this book, you will notice a significant improvement in your sport performance. The power of nutrition is strong and is often the limiter for athletes in competing well. Until now. Welcome to the future of sports nutrition.

1

Energy Systems and Physical Periodization

It may seem odd to begin a sports nutrition book with discussions of energy systems and the concept of physical periodization, but both of them provide a staple in your foundational knowledge of understanding how to use and change your nutrition throughout your training. By knowing about the various energy systems in your body that are called upon during different types of exercise, you will have a much better idea of which nutrients are being used and which are not in your training sessions. If you do not have a clear idea of your physical goals associated with each training cycle, you miss the opportunities to implement specific nutrition strategies that optimize your health and performance.

ENERGY SYSTEMS

The body's three energy systems that provide you with the energy to fuel your training sessions—from warm-ups to sprints to strength training to long endurance training—are the phosphagen system, the glycolytic system, and the aerobic pathway. These systems are engaged at different times and in different amounts based on the intensity and duration of training. Warm-ups exert a much different metabolic response and energy system demand on the body than does sprinting. Strength and power training are somewhat different than long endurance training. It is these alterations in training load (volume and intensity) that dictate what, when, and how your energy systems contribute to fueling your workouts. The carbohydrates, protein, and fat that you eat on a daily basis and store in your body follow different metabolic paths, and their utilization depends on the intensity and duration of your training.

The phosphagen system, also known as the phosphocreatine or creatine phosphate system, is an anaerobic (without oxygen) pathway that supplies immediate energy to your working muscles. The amount of phosphocreatine stored in your body is limited, so this system only provides you enough energy for about 10 seconds of high-intensity exercise. Many sprint and explosive power athletes utilize this system. After the initial 10 seconds of this type of training, athletes typically require about 2–4 minutes of rest to allow regeneration of the phosphocreatine used. It is very important for athletes participating in this type of training to allow this rest interval between sets to allow the energy system to recovery during this maximal energy use.

The glycolytic system, also known as glycolysis, is another anaerobic metabolic pathway that functions to break down glucose or glycogen to energy. As with the first energy system, the glycolytic system also has limited stores and provides only enough fuel for about 1–2 minutes of high-intensity exercise. This system also yields lactate molecules, which can be thought of as friends rather than foes. Lactate can be used as an energy source to fuel your muscles at certain intensity levels.

The third energy system, aerobic energy, uses oxygen to provide energy and can thus produce a larger amount of energy. Pyruvate, a product of glycolysis, enters the mitochondria (the energy factories of the cell) and generates a constant supply of energy to fuel working muscles for hours and hours.

When you first begin exercise with a bout of lower-intensity cardiovascular exercise or a dynamic warm-up, your body utilizes primarily anaerobic systems, with a small contribution from the aerobic pathway. As you progress into more aerobic exercise, your body calls upon more of the aerobic energy system, with less contribution from the anaerobic energy systems. As a general rule, high-intensity and maximal training rely more on anaerobic metabolism, whereas lower-intensity and longer-duration training rely more on aerobic metabolism. Very rarely does one energy system perform all of the work at any given point throughout exercise.

PHYSICAL PERIODIZATION

Periodization is a strategy that promotes improvement in performance by providing varied training specificity, intensity, and volume in training sessions throughout the year. By manipulating each of these variables with just the right blend of science and art, you can almost guarantee an improvement in performance.

Figure 1.1 depicts physical periodization in a graphic form. As you can see, there are three main cycles: macrocycle, mesocycle, and microcycle. Each of these cycles have very specific physical goals. The macrocycle is normally defined as the big picture and

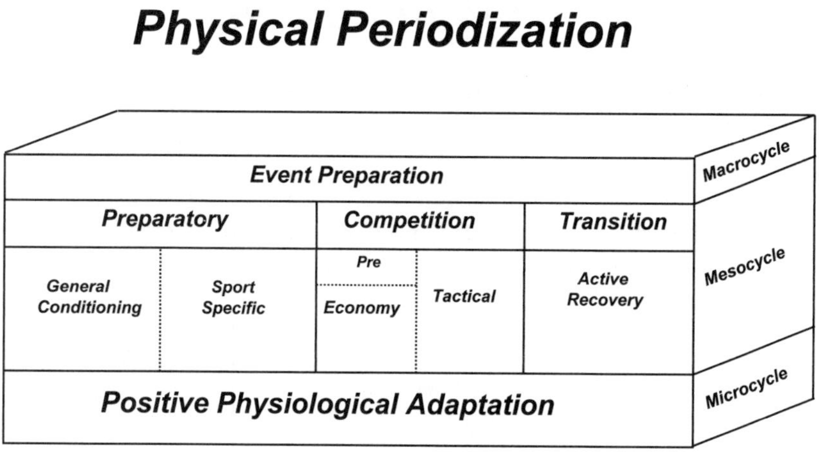

Physical Periodization

Event Preparation					Macrocycle
Preparatory		Competition		Transition	Mesocycle
General Conditioning	Sport Specific	Pre Economy	Tactical	Active Recovery	
Positive Physiological Adaptation					Microcycle

Figure 1.1

includes the entire year (annual training plan) or 4-year plan (for Olympic athletes). The mesocycle is a smaller portion of time than the macrocycle and typically spans 2–3 months. Each mesocycle is typically separated into three specific subcategories, which include the pre-season or base, in-season or competition, and off-season or transition. Each of the mesocycle subcategories has its own very specific physical goals based on the status of the athlete and competition frequency and duration.

General and sport-specific conditioning are included in the pre-season, and the physical goals are a result of the type of athlete, sport, and developmental stage. For example, many less-experienced endurance athletes may have goals of improving aerobic endurance, strength, and flexibility, whereas more-experienced athletes may try to improve anaerobic endurance, power, and economy. Strength, power, and team-sport athletes use this time of the training year to develop good technique, foundational strength, and movement patterns to build a strong body that is ready for more intense training in the next cycle. (See Figure 1.2, Periodization Boxes.) During the in-season, many athletes are getting ready

Training Cycles

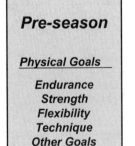

Pre-season	In-Season	Off-Season
Physical Goals	*Physical Goals*	*Physical Goals*
Endurance	*Speed*	*Recovery*
Strength	*Economy*	*Prehab*
Flexibility	*Skills*	*Rehab*
Technique	*Power*	*Fun*
Other Goals	*Other Goals*	*Other Goals*

Figure 1.2

for competition by training to improve competition specific strength, force, economy, skills, power, and speed.

During the off-season, most athletes take a reprieve from structured training—for a few days to a few weeks—with goals consisting of rehabilitation, recovery, and enjoying a small amount of time without formal training.

Each sport has varying lengths of each cycle. Much of this is dependent on the competition cycle of the sport. In many sports, athletes compete year-round, with very little down time and a nonexistent off-season (e.g., sailing). Other sports follow specific seasons, and athletes have scheduled recovery in between the competition season and the pre-season (e.g., football, soccer, triathlon). But it is always important to realize the competition demands and structure of your sport. Once you have this information, you can easily build a physical periodization plan that accommodates your goals and progression in sport.

HISTORY OF PERIODIZATION

The concept of periodization dates back to the ancient Olympic Games and was introduced in a more structured manner in the 1940s, when Soviet sports scientists discovered that athletic performance was improved by varying the training stresses throughout the year rather than by maintaining the same training from month to month. This led to the formal division of an athlete's year into cycles, with differing training stresses. The East Germans and Romanians further developed this concept by applying goals to the various cycles.

There are many models of periodization, but I have chosen two specific models that are opposites in the planning and implementation processes and that provide you with an idea of different approaches in attempting to attain the same overall goal of improved performance. An understanding of these two foundational models assists you with understanding and implementing nutrition principles to support your training load changes.

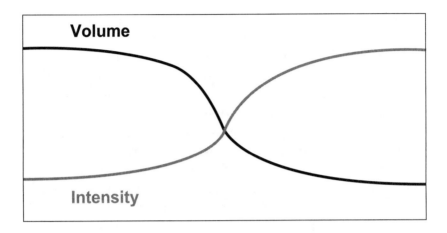

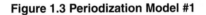

Figure 1.3 Periodization Model #1

The first popular periodization model (Figure 1.3) follows the concept that training should begin with a general physical preparation phase in which volume is moderate and intensity is low. The intention is to develop strong tendons and ligaments, build strength, and begin to improve cardiovascular fitness. Many athletes and coaches explain this type of preparation in terms of the foundation of a house: the concrete must be poured before framing the walls.

As training continues in this model, volume is typically reduced to allow the intensity of training to increase in a sport-specific manner. More time is spent practicing specific sport skills. Many novice to intermediate level athletes have great success with this type of periodization model because they are still in the developmental stages of sport progression. The competition season can be quite demanding, with frequent competitions and very little opportunities to train.

Once the competition season is complete, both volume and intensity are reduced to allow the athlete to recover. This type of pattern is also experienced during the initial phases of injury, when a nutritional shift is required to support the injury status.

There is another common model used by athletes and coaches that employs the exact opposite concept of the first model. As you

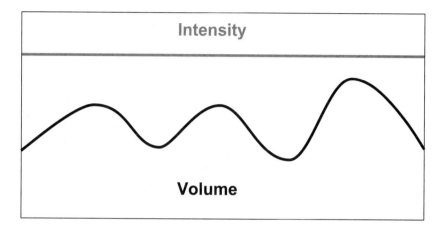

Figure 1.4 Periodization Model #2

can see in figure 1.4, volume and intensity do not cross, and intensity is maintained at a high level throughout the training program. The volume of training fluctuates in response to competitions. This method is more commonly used with elite athletes who have at least 10 years of sport experience. Because the intensity is maintained at a high level, there is more risk of injury and overtraining. This method is often needed for more experienced athletes, however, because it provides them with the necessary stimulus for performance enhancement that the previous model does not provide.

It is very common for athletes to fluctuate between both periodization methods at different points in their careers and even during a training year because their sport and their body may require different stimuli and, more important, different recovery methods to achieve optimal performance.

Regardless of which periodization method is used, it is important to understand the differences in energy utilization and expenditure, which have a direct impact on your nutrition periodization program (as described in the following chapter). Maintaining a high intensity of training throughout your training year requires different macronutrient shifts than do frequent volume and intensity shifts.

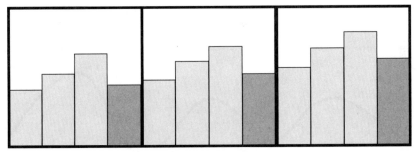

Standard

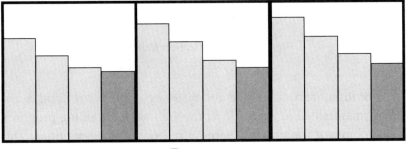

Reverse

Figure 1.5 Traditional and Reverse Periodization Models

Other types of periodization that fall into the previously mentioned models include traditional and reverse periodization. As you can see in Figure 1.5, a generic model of traditional (standard) periodization is characterized with a progressive increase in load (volume and intensity) over weeks to months. In this example, each block represents one week, so you see a three-week build to one-week recovery cycle. Reverse periodization is the opposite and begins with a higher training load with progressive decreases in load. As mentioned previously, traditional periodization is used quite frequently with novice to intermediate athletes, whereas reverse periodization is more commonly used with advanced athletes. Of course, these two types of periodization can also be used together in an athlete's training year. The important point from a nutrition perspective is, again, to note the changes in volume and intensity, because these institute a change in the nutrition program.

There are many principles associated with periodization, and the science can be somewhat confusing. If you have a basic understanding of periodization, you can use it in the development and implementation of your specific training program. The most important thing to remember is that each cycle should be constructed to have a set of specific physiological, psychological, and nutritional goals that help you improve as an athlete. As long as you progress in a steady, logical way, making sure that your body is prepared for each cycle, you should be more than ready to compete to your potential season after season.

PROACTIVE VS. REACTIVE PERIODIZATION

The difference between proactive and reactive periodization is simply that the former allows you to plan your recovery and rejuvenation ahead of time, so that you improve performance, whereas the latter does not promote an increase in fitness, because you may always be reacting to your training sessions. The hard truth is that if you go weeks or months without planned rest, you cannot reach your full potential. Athletes know their bodies better than anyone, but it is often difficult for them to step outside their bodies and provide an objective assessment of their fatigue scale. Because you may not be 100% accurate in your assessment, it is important to structure planned and frequent rest into your training stressors. This rest can range from a day of light stretching to a complete rest day or a block of rest days in a row. No matter which method you choose, the important message is to try to predict closely when your body needs rest rather than forcing it to rest because you were not able to train hard during a workout, make certain times, or master technical skills.

Recovery is extremely crucial to your success as an athlete. Not many athletes realize that during cycles of high volume and intensity,

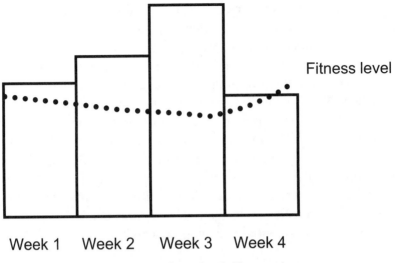

Fitness level

Week 1   Week 2   Week 3   Week 4

Figure 1.6 One-month Mesocycle

fitness level does not improve. In fact, it may actually decrease as a result of the repeated physical stress placed on the body. It is only during planned recovery, which includes less volume and intensity, that the body actually improves its fitness. Quite simply, if you allow your body to rest and repair the damage that you did to it during training, you get stronger, faster, and more powerful.

To further illustrate this point, Figure 1.6 provides an example of a one-month mesocycle in which training volume is steadily increased each week, which is typical for athletes following a traditional periodization model. You can see that as volume increases, fitness level slowly starts to decrease. As soon as the recovery week begins, however, the body rejuvenates itself and recovers from the previous three weeks of training. The result is an increase in fitness.

By following a model that focuses on proactive periodization and recovery, you can reap the rewards of improved performance without injury or overtraining. It does not matter which recovery method or system you choose. The important thing is that you make recovery a priority. Take a day, a week, or a month for recovery, but be sure to include it during times of high volume and/or intensity. Remember, recovery is needed in order for your body to improve. Also, be sure to account for other stressors or time commitments that increase your stress, such as career, family, travel, or social engagements. Although it may not seem apparent, these add to your overall training load stress response and should be minimized when your physical training load is high in order to ensure a faster recovery from training.

OVERTRAINING (UNDERRECOVERY) AND INJURY

Overtraining, also known as underrecovery, and injury are common among athletes. Whether you are just beginning your athletic career, if you are an Olympic medalist, you are likely to fall victim to one of these at some point in your athletic career. Following a well-periodized training program is extremely important in the prevention of underrecovery or injury, but their occurrence may sometimes be out of your control.

If you choose to follow a less periodized, more random training program, you may subject yourself to a higher risk of overtraining and injury. This could result in an unplanned break or, quite possibly, in forfeiting your entire competitive season. Properly planned recovery becomes extremely important during training, whether it is recovery days, weeks, or cycles. There is a limit to your capacity to endure and adapt to intense training. Once this threshold is crossed, your body fails to adapt and your performance declines rapidly. In fact, 10–20% of athletes who train intensively may fall prey to overtraining at some point during their sport career.

The term "overtraining" itself is fraught with controversy and confusion. The following definitions are commonly used when discussing overtraining:

Overload:　　　A planned, systematic, and progressive increase in training, with the goal of improving performance.

Overreaching: An unplanned, excessive overload in training,
                   with inadequate rest. Poor performance is
                   observed in training and competition.

Overtraining: Untreated overreaching that results in
                   chronic decreases in performance and
                   impaired ability to train. This may require
                   medical attention.

There are many causes associated with overtraining, but the primary cause is a poorly planned training program. The main culprit is a rapid increase in training volume and intensity, combined with inadequate recovery and rest. Other types of stressors, such as competitions, environmental factors, psychosocial factors, improper nutrition, and travel, can increase the stress of training and contribute to overtraining.

If you find yourself fitting into one of the categories of overreaching or overtraining, the smartest thing to do is rest. Recovery may take days, weeks, or even months, but unstructured activity is the best remedy to help you recover and get back in condition to train. In most cases, if overreaching is caught early, you do not have to stop training completely; you only need to reduce training volume and intensity.

SIGNS OF OVERTRAINING

It is extremely important to recognize the signs of overtraining before it becomes too severe. The physical signs of overtraining include the following:

- Decreased performance
- Loss of coordination
- Prolonged recovery
- Elevated morning heart rate
- Headaches
- Loss of appetite

- Muscle soreness/tenderness
- Gastrointestinal disturbances
- Decreased ability to ward off infection

There are also nonphysical symptoms, such as the following:

- Depression
- Apathy
- Difficulty concentrating
- Emotional sensitivity
- Decreased self-esteem

I highly recommend that you keep a watchful eye on your daily health and physical adaptations of training in order to prevent overtraining. Once you become overtrained, it is nearly impossible to heal within 6–12 months, which could mean the loss of an entire competitive season. Smart training with good recovery is the key to preventing overtraining.

As well as providing you with the energy you need to train hard, proper nutrition can help you avoid overtraining, and it can speed recovery. The next chapter addresses in detail how your nutrition plan can complement your periodization program. Training and eating appropriately help you become a better and healthier athlete, regardless of your sport, age, or athletic goals.

2

Nutrients for Life

This chapter provides in-depth knowledge of the six essential nutrients so that you have a better understanding of how these nutrients interact in your body and support your physical training needs. It also gives you the information required for you to recognize why certain nutrients are better than others during certain times of your training year. In addition, you will learn the intricacies of each nutrient class and the distinct differences among them, all of which affect your health and performance as it relates to sport and your application of nutrition periodization to your training program.

THE SIX ESSENTIAL NUTRIENTS

The six essential nutrients that the body requires in order to maintain life and support training are the following:

1. Carbohydrates
2. Protein
3. Fat
4. Water
5. Vitamins
6. Minerals

Before explaining the details of each nutrient, I provide an overview of the digestive system, because gastrointestinal (GI) disturbances are common among athletes. Having a good knowledge of how foods pass through your system may help you better prepare your digestive system for competition and prevent GI distress in the future.

DIGESTION BASICS

After you eat or drink something, your brain and body release hormones that direct the digestive system to digest and absorb the foodstuff. The digestive system itself is a flexible, muscular tube extending from the mouth through the throat, esophagus, stomach, small intestine, large intestine, and rectum to the anus. It has a total length of about 26 feet. It is a highly specialized organ that is designed to convert food into nourishment for your cells, protect you from invading organisms and toxins, and dispose of a large variety of waste products.

The digestive tract is composed of the following organs with their roles:

- Mouth: chews and mixes food with saliva, which moistens the food to make it easier to swallow. Salivary amylase, a digestive enzyme in the mouth, begins the process of carbohydrate metabolism.

- Esophagus: passes food to the stomach. Peristalsis, a series of rhythmic contractions in the esophageal wall, moves the food down the tube, which takes 4–10 seconds. At the end of the esophagus, a muscular ring, the lower esophageal sphincter, opens and lets the food enter the stomach.

- Stomach: adds acid, enzymes, and fluid; churns, mixes, and grinds food to a liquid mass. Once food enters the stomach, muscles begin to churn and mix the food with acids and enzymes in order to break down the food into smaller, more digestible pieces. Cells in the stomach lining secrete mucus, hydrochloric acid, and pepsin, which aid in this process. Most nutrients, except for water, salt, sugars, and alcohol, still need to be digested further. Once the food has been turned into the thick liquid chyme, it is stored at the bottom of the stomach; once it becomes the proper consistency, a muscle between the stomach and small intestine opens to allow the chyme to enter the small intestine.

- Small intestine: secretes enzymes that digest carbohydrates, fat, and protein; absorbs nutrients into the blood. Chyme secreted from the stomach moves down into the small intestine.

  Digestion of chyme continues as it is further broken down in the small intestine until the nutrients can be absorbed by millions of villi, finger-like projections covering the wall of the small intestine, into the bloodstream.

- Large intestine or colon: reabsorbs water and minerals; passes waste and some water to the rectum. Undigested food and some water enter the large intestine, which removes water from undigested nutrients.

- Rectum: stores waste prior to elimination.

- Anus: holds rectum closed; opens to allow elimination.

The digestive tract also has the following accessory organs that aid in digestion:

- Salivary glands: donate a starch-digesting enzyme and a trace of fat-digesting enzyme.
- Liver: manufactures bile that helps break down fat.
- Gallbladder: stores bile until it is needed.
- Bile duct: carries the bile to the small intestine.
- Pancreatic duct: carries pancreatic juice to the small intestine.
- Pancreas: manufactures enzymes to digest all energy-yielding nutrients and releases bicarbonate, which neutralizes stomach acid that enters the small intestine.

It usually takes 6–8 hours after you eat before food passes through your stomach and small intestine, depending on the size and composition of the snack or meal. Removal of food residue from the large intestine usually begins after 24 hours; it can take up to 72 hours from entry to exit. Interestingly, anything inside your digestive tract is not technically inside your body. Food must be broken down and pass through the intestinal wall before it becomes inside your body once again.

The digestive system is so specialized that it even has its own nervous system and quite a significant immune system to keep it

---

FUELTIP

Prebiotics and probiotics have become quite popular among athletes and with good reason. Both have positive health effects on the digestive system by restoring the balance of bacteria in the digestive tract. Prebiotics are indigestible food ingredients that beneficially affect the host by selectively stimulating the growth of one or a limited number of bacterial species in the colon. In simpler terms, they are the "food" for the beneficial bacteria in your gut. Probiotics (good bacteria) are live microbial food ingredients that exert health benefits. Two of the most common probiotics are acidophilus and bifidobacteria, which can be found in foods such as yogurt and sauerkraut.

If a positive balance of good bacteria is maintained, the bad bacteria are less able to produce problems for your system. The benefits of probiotics include inhibiting the growth of bacteria that cause disease, synthesizing B vitamins, increasing the availability of nutrients, decreasing symptoms of gastroesophageal reflux disease (GERD) and lactose intolerance, and boosting the immune system.

Prebiotics are extremely beneficial in promoting good gut health because they nourish probiotics to help them grow. Prebiotics are often found in oligosaccharides; common food sources include fruits, legumes, whole grains, garlic, and onions.

Probiotic supplements are common in the marketplace and can be found as powders, wafers, liquids, and capsules. They are often expressed in billions of live organisms: a typical dose is 3–5 billion live organisms.

healthy. In fact, the largest part of the immune system is inside the digestive tract lining.

The immune system in the digestive system is important in helping the intestines respond to injury from bad bacteria, toxins, parasites, and viruses. Your immune system has to determine whether or not to develop a tolerance to food that you put into your mouth. Your immune system typically accepts most foods; its ability to make these decisions depends largely on the balance of good bacteria that you have inside your intestinal tract.

When your digestive tract's immune system does not like what you ate, however, it attacks the food by increasing inflammation and mucus production. Inflammation of the digestive tube can lead to damage of the lining.

Trillions of bacteria live in your digestive tract. Although this may sound alarming, some of these are very good bacteria that are needed to protect against invading organisms, to protect you by working with the immune system, to create vitamins, and to break down food that you eat.

Transit Time in the Gut

Because so much can go wrong when you are consuming calories before, during, and after training and competition, it is important for athletes to time the quantity and quality of food eaten properly in order to supply enough fuel for the working muscles and brain without experiencing GI concerns. Some athletes have the luxury of eating a snack or meal before a training session, but others are forced to wait until afterwards because of an early morning start or their body's inability to handle food or beverage in the minutes to hours before a quality workout.

There is normal variability among transit time through the GI tract, which can be significantly affected by the composition of the meal and the psychological stress of the situation. During competition, the stress response is elevated, which can induce a negative effect on the processing of food and beverages.

Research studies have proved that all substances do not move through the GI system at the same rate and that they do not always leave in the same order as they arrive as a result of the interactions of body processes breaking down the food as it travels throughout the digestive tract. Although there has been much research on this topic, it is still difficult to pinpoint how long the food that you eat before a workout or competition actually takes to become fully digested from the stomach, used in the small intestine, and excreted through the large intestine. The variables are far too many to make an generalized statement, but Table 2.1 provides rough estimates of the time that it takes for solid, mixed-nutrient foods to move through your system, which allows you to better plan for your pre-workout snack or meal.

The volume of food and liquid that you eat also influences the rate at which they empty from the stomach. For example, if you drink a glass of water, your stomach becomes distended, but, because there are no solids to be ground or liquefied, your stomach gets off easy, and so it does not have to do any additional processing of the water before it is absorbed in the small intestine. Therefore, the rate of gastric emptying is fast. If you eat a mixed meal such as a turkey sandwich with an apple, your stomach again becomes distended. The solid food, however, needs to be broken down by enzymes and stomach acid and is therefore not allowed to enter the small intestine at a high rate to prevent overload. This leads to slower gastric emptying.

After you consume a normal, solid meal, minimal gastric emptying continues for up to 30 minutes, which is then followed by a linear increase of emptying. For liquid meals, it is quite the opposite. They are usually emptied immediately. The main factor

Table 2.1
Transit Times of Food

Complete emptying of the stomach	4 to 5 hours
Complete emptying of the small intestine	5 to 6 hours
Transit through the colon	30–40 hours

in how quickly a liquid or liquid meal is emptied from the stomach, however, is volume. Larger volumes of liquid empty more quickly than smaller volumes.

FUELTIP

Most athletes, for some reason or another, think that sipping on a sports drink delivers nutrients in a more "time-released" manner. In fact, the opposite is true. If you sip on a sports drink, it does not exit the stomach quickly, which means that it is not delivered to the small intestine where it can be used. Gulps are better than sips.

For most athletes I recommend more liquid or semi-solid calorie sources because those have a shorter transit time. The quicker that nutrients can exit your stomach, the faster they can enter the small intestine and be absorbed and used by your body. If you have early morning practices or workouts, choose smoothies, sports drinks, or juices.

FUELTIP

Remember that you should not overconsume calories before a training session or competition because a large meal slows digestion. If at all possible, begin your eating preparation at least 2–4 hours before the start of training. If this is not possible, it is still important to consume some calories, even in smaller amounts. Athletes who have early morning practices or competitions (or more than two workouts in a day with less than 2 hours in between) are challenged even more. Keep in mind that upon waking from your overnight fast, you can be as much as 3% dehydrated and lose as much as 40% of your glycogen (stored carbohydrate) stores. Although I consider these percentages to be a bit on the extreme side, the point is that you wake up in a somewhat dehydrated and malnourished state. Your body needs fluids and calories before you begin higher-intensity or longer-duration exercise. It may not be as important to fuel for shorter, more aerobically based training in the morning as long as a feeding can be planned immediately afterward.

Now that you have a good understanding of how food moves through your body, let me discuss each of the nutrients that your body requires to sustain life and a high level of sport performance.

CARBOHYDRATES

Carbohydrates are the ultimate source of energy for your body and your brain. In fact, your brain relies primarily on glucose to function properly. For athletes competing in sports where cognitive function and mental focus and concentration are important (almost every sport I know of), supplying the body with enough foods that are rich in carbohydrates is crucial. Carbohydrates are vital to athletes because of their ability to maintain energy levels and high mental functioning.

In addition to providing energy, carbohydrates also play a protein-sparing role. When glycogen levels become low, the body begins to make glucose from protein and fat, although these are very inefficient processes and most use energy to make a small amount of energy. Although this process may sound positive, it can be detrimental. Almost every athlete met wants to maintain or improve lean muscle mass. If your body turns to your protein stores to make glucose to fuel your brain, where does it come from first? It comes from your lean muscle stores.

Each gram of carbohydrate provides four calories. Depending on your gender and size, you can only store approximately 1,400–1,800 calories from carbohydrates in your muscles, liver, and blood (refer to Table 2.2). The digestion of carbohydrates begins in the mouth, as mentioned previously, and then passes through the stomach to the small intestine. It is in the small intestine that all carbohydrates (except fiber) enter the bloodstream and are sent to the liver for further breakdown and delivery to the cells or to be stored as glycogen.

Table 2.2
Storage Amounts of Carbohydrates in the Body

Source	Storage Form	Total Body Calories
Carbohydrate	Serum glucose	20
	Liver glycogen	400
	Muscle glycogen	1,500

TYPES OF CARBOHYDRATES

There are two main classifications of carbohydrates: simple and complex, each with different chemical structures.

Simple carbohydrates, often called simple sugars, are made up of short chains of sugars and are classified as mono-, di-, and oligosaccharides. Complex carbohydrates, or complex sugars, are made up of longer chains, also called polysaccharides, which include starch and fiber. In general terms, as a sugar becomes more complex, it is more difficult to digest and its digestion takes longer.

Monosaccharides, which include glucose, fructose, and galactose, are the simplest form of carbohydrate. They are made up of one simple sugar molecule and are the easiest to digest.

FUELTIP

Glucose is the main carbohydrate found in the blood and is used to make the glycogen stored in the liver and muscles. Fructose is the simple sugar found in fruit and honey and is sweeter than common table sugar. It is digested more slowly because it must first pass through the liver to be broken down into glucose. Galactose does not directly stimulate an insulin response; similar to fructose, it must first visit the liver to be broken down into glucose. Agave nectar, mostly comprised of fructose, is a natural liquid sweetener extracted from the agave plant. It does not spike your blood sugar levels and is absorbed more slowly in your body.

Disaccharides include sucrose (glucose + fructose), lactose (glucose + galactose), and maltose (glucose + glucose). These are made up of two monosaccharides and are not as easy to digest as monosaccharides.

FUELTIP

Sucrose is extracted from sugar cane and beet sugar and is the most common disaccharide in the diet. Honey is primarily a combination of the natural sugars fructose and glucose (38% and 31%, respectively). The third major component of honey is water, accounting for approximately 17%. Honey is a natural sweetener and is typically easy to digest but takes longer to get into the bloodstream.

Oligosaccharides, by definition, contain three to nine monosaccharides and include maltodextrins, corn syrup, and high-fructose corn syrup and are most often manufactured. Artificially sweetened foods often contain oligosaccharides. These take longer to digest than either mono- or disaccharides.

FUELTIP

High-fructose corn syrup is an especially sweet corn syrup. It differs from traditional corn syrup in that 45–55% of its carbohydrate is enzymatically hydrolyzed to the simple sugars glucose and fructose. It is less viscous than traditional corn syrup but has nearly twice the concentration of mono- and disaccharides compared with regular corn syrup. It is the predominant sweetener found in commercially sweetened foods.

Complex Carbohydrates

Polysaccharides are often referred to as complex carbohydrates and include starch and fiber. They are made up of long, complex chains of sugars and require more complex mechanisms for digestion than simple carbohydrates, which extends their time to be digested.

FUELTIP

Glucose polymers are not as sweet as sucrose or corn syrup and provide a greater amount of energy without being too sweet. Maltodextrin is a glucose polymer and is often found in processed foods. Brown rice syrup is a polysaccharide and is digested and released into the bloodstream more slowly than simple sugars. It is a thick amber syrup made by combining sprouted barley with cooked brown rice and fermenting it in a warm environment.

High Molecular Weight Carbohydrates

Blood glucose concentrations are influenced by the movement of glucose from the stomach to the intestine and finally into the blood. This becomes important because the osmolality of a solution has been shown to influence the gastric emptying rate from the stomach. Carbohydrate sources with high osmolality may delay glucose transportation by slowing gastric emptying. A steady supply of glucose without much delay of delivery to the blood and to the working muscles and brain is ideal to maintain physical and cognitive functioning.

High molecular weight (HMW) carbohydrates, polyglucosides or glucose polymers, have a low osmolality, which makes their entry and exit time in and out of the stomach quick and efficient. The opposite is true for low molecular weight (LMW) carbohydrates, which tend to increase the entry and exit time in and out of the stomach because of their higher osmolality. An inverse relationship exists between the molecular weight and gastric emptying time.

Sugar Alcohols

Another class of carbohydrates that is important to understand are sugar alcohols, also known as polyols. You may see them advertised as "zero impact carbs" or "net carbs." Sugar alcohols are ingredients used as sweeteners and bulking agents and occur naturally in foods such as fruits and berries. As a sugar substitute, they provide fewer calories (about one-half to one-third fewer calories) than regular sugar. This is because they are converted to glucose more slowly, require little or no insulin to be metabolized, and don't cause sudden increases in blood sugar.

FUELTIP

If you see a product that uses the term "sugar free" or "no added sugar," it must list the total grams of sugar alcohols on the nutrition label. Common sugar alcohols include mannitol, sorbitol, xylitol, lactitol, isomalt, maltitol, and hydrogenated starch hydrolysates (HSH).

The popularity of sugar alcohols is based on their being fewer calories in these products; they are of particular interest to athletes seeking weight loss. Some athletes, however, may experience consequences associated with eating products containing sugar alcohols. The most common side effects include the possibilities of bloating and diarrhea, both of which can have a negative impact on training and performance. So be sure to check the nutrition facts label and the ingredients list of food products for sugar alcohols. If you choose to use these products, do so in a training cycle where you can afford to have a GI challenge without it affecting your performance. You need to determine whether these products do or do not work for your particular body. And do not consume too many sugar alcohols at one time.

Glycemic Response

Each sugar has a different glycemic index value, which means that it is digested faster or slower. Choosing the wrong sports nutrition product based on its sugar profile has the potential to cause serious stomach problems. The glycemic index of foods can be affected by many different variables, such as preparation method, protein and fat presence, fiber content, and more. It is very rare to find a food that has only one sugar in it that is not influenced by the other factors that affect its glycemic index value.

The glycemic response (GR) of a food is a measure of that food's ability to raise blood sugar. The two main components in determining GR are the food's glycemic index and its glycemic load (GL). Many athletes have, at some point in their training, adopted the use of the glycemic index, but, unfortunately, the GL is not often being used in conjunction with it; therefore, the athlete is plagued with misinformation and is using only one-half of the equation. Let me discuss this in more detail so that you can understand what using the overall GR means from a realistic standpoint.

Glycemic Index

The glycemic index has existed for quite some time, but its popularity seems to ebb and flow based on which fad diet is most popular. Simply put, the glycemic index is a standard measure of how quickly 50 grams of a particular food's carbohydrates are converted to sugar and thus affect your blood sugar over a 2-hour period.

Remember, simple carbohydrates contain only one or two sugar units in a chain, whereas complex carbohydrates contain hundreds to thousands of sugar units in a single chain. In the past, simple carbohydrates were classified as having a high glycemic index, that is, as causing a quick rise and fall in blood sugar, whereas complex carbohydrates were classified as providing sustained energy, with a more gentle rise in blood sugar. In terms of the glycemic index, simple carbohydrates were classified as "bad" and complex carbohydrates as "good."

Even though this notion may seem fairly logical, recent data indicate that this concept is out of date. Nonrefined or wholesome carbohydrates are always preferred because they provide important nutrients, whereas refined carbohydrates do not and therefore should be limited in your daily nutrition plan. Many athletes, however, correlate "wholesome" with complex and "simple" with refined, which is simply not the case. For example, fruit is considered a simple carbohydrate, but these carbohydrates are unrefined, and fruit is very nutrient-dense, meaning that it has many vitamins and minerals and a good amount of fiber. It has been shown that each food produces its own blood sugar profile; there is not a strong correlation to whether or not it contains simple or complex carbohydrates. Some complex carbohydrates can be digested, absorbed, and utilized as quickly as simple sugars, meaning that they have similar GR.

The following is a short list of factors that can affect the glycemic index of foods:

- Biochemical structure of the carbohydrate
- Absorption process
- Size of meal
- Degree of processing
- Contents and timing of previous meal
- Fat, fiber, and protein content
- Ripeness

You can see that the glycemic index of a carbohydrate is dependent upon many factors other than just the structure of the carbohydrate. It is impossible to classify a food as "healthy" or "unhealthy" simply based on its complex or simple chemical structure or based solely on its glycemic index. The glycemic index tells you how fast a carbohydrate increases your blood sugar levels, but it does not tell you how much of that carbohydrate is in a serving of that food. This is where the GL comes into play. Both the glycemic index and the GL are needed to determine the GR that a given food has on your body.

GL

GL is the numerical value of the glycemic index divided by 100 and multiplied by the food's available carbohydrate content in grams. GL takes the glycemic index into account but is based on how much carbohydrate is in the food or drink. The GL is numerically lower than the glycemic index (see Table 2.3).

Table 2.3
Glycemic Index and Glycemic Load Numerical Classification

Value	Glycemic Index	GL
High	≥70	20
Medium	56–69	11–19
Low	≤55	≤10

Here is an example of GL.

• Watermelon has a glycemic index of 72. A recommended serving of ½ cup is 4 ounces or 120 grams of watermelon. This serving has 6 grams of carbohydrates.

• To calculate the GL, divide the glycemic index by 100 and multiply by carbohydrate content in grams:

$(72/100) \times 6 = 4.32$, or 4 when rounded.

In this example, a food with a high glycemic index becomes a food with a low GL. Thus, based on the serving size and quantity eaten, watermelon has a better GR and therefore results in a lower rise in blood sugar than its glycemic index indicates. Keep in mind that as you increase the serving size eaten, you increase the amount of carbohydrates eaten, which in turn increases the GR of the food.

In many cases, GL is not based on a typical amount of food eaten, so GL does not provide realistic information unless the food is weighed prior to consuming it. I am certainly not suggesting that you weigh all of your food before eating it, which would soon become quite a monotonous task. The important take-home lesson about GL is that it provides an understanding of the relationship between a specific amount of food and its biochemical response.

Let's look at another example. The glycemic index of ice cream is 37 and the GL is 4, based on consumption of 50 grams of ice cream. Sixty-five grams of ice cream equals ½ cup, so 50 grams of ice cream is less than ½ cup. Realistically, who eats less than ½ cup of ice cream at a time? As the serving size increases, so does the GR.

In this complex but informative section about GR, I hope I have accomplished three goals:

1. Provided you with enough information for you to consider factoring in the concept of GR as you design your personal nutrition plan.
2. Proved to you that using glycemic index or GL by itself is not useful and that the two concepts must be considered together.
3. Illustrated that, although the GR of foods is important, it is not mandatory that you follow it with all of your meals all of the time. Following the basic nutrition recommendations of eating fruits and vegetables, whole grains, lean meats, and foods containing healthy fats and reducing the amount of refined foods should always be your focus. Food is fun and is an important part of your life. Don't get caught up in calculating the glycemic index for every meal you eat, as that will detract from some of the enjoyment that food provides in your life.

Carbohydrate Food Sources

It may seem obvious, but, because of the introduction of many new foods to the market, there is sometimes confusion regarding which foods are classified as carbohydrates. In brief, any food that is made from rice, oats, wheat, barley, cornmeal, or a cereal grain is considered a grain product or carbohydrate. Grains are not created always equally, however. Grains are divided into whole grains and refined grains.

Whole grains contain the entire grain kernel, which includes the bran, germ, and endosperm. Foods such as whole-wheat flour, oatmeal (not the instant packaged type), whole cornmeal, bulgur, and brown rice can be classified as whole grains. In contrast, refined grains are milled, which is a process that removes the bran and germ. Although this improves the shelf life of

Table 2.4
Types of Grains

Whole Grains	Refined Grains*
Brown rice	Cornbread
Buckwheat	Crackers
Bulgur	Couscous
Oatmeal (rolled or stone cut oats)	Corn tortillas
Muesli	Noodles
Whole grain barley	Grits
Whole-wheat bread, pasta, crackers, tortillas, rolls	Pasta
Wild rice	Pita bread
Whole rye	Pretzels
Amaranth	White bread, rolls
Millet	White rice
Quinoa	
Sorghum	
Triticale	

*Some refined grain food products may be made from whole grains. Be sure to check the ingredient list and look for the words "whole wheat" or "whole grain" to decide whether they are whole grain sources of carbohydrates.

products, it removes the beneficial nutrients, including fiber, iron, and many B vitamins. Foods such as white flour, bread, and rice are classified as refined grains. Because these are stripped of some nutrients, they are often enriched, which means that nutrients such as the B vitamins, thiamin, riboflavin, niacin, and folic acid, along with iron, are added back into the refined grain after processing.

Fruits and vegetables are also rich sources of carbohydrates and provide a significant amount of vitamins and minerals. They are best in their natural state, so that the fiber, vitamins, and minerals are present in high amounts. Frozen fruits and vegetables are a close second to fresh and are very easy to have on hand as long as you have a freezer. In fact, if cooked properly, frozen varieties maintain much of their nutrients, similar to fresh. Frozen fruits and vegetables make for great stir fry dishes, fruit smoothies, and are sometimes cheaper per ounce than fresh. In addition, they can be stored longer and therefor do not require frequent trips to the grocery store. I often recommend frozen fruits and vegetables to athletes because it is just a fact of life that busy schedules predominate and your ability to visit the grocery store frequently to buy fresh fruits and vegetables is often limited. Keep a few bags of different varieties of fruits and vegetables in your freezer and you will find it easier to meet your daily serving recommendations.

FUELTIP

Frozen fruits are staples to have in your freezer for that pre- or post-workout fruit smoothie. Simply put one cup of skim, soy, almond, or rice milk in a blender with one cup of frozen fruit, and you have a very well-balanced snack that will fuel your body before your workout or begin the nutrition recovery process after your workout.

Dairy products, nuts, legumes, and soy products are also good sources of carbohydrates. Be sure to choose lower fat options of dairy products. Even though nuts are rich in carbohydrates, they are also high in fat, albeit more of the healthy fat, but, nonetheless, they are high calorie foods. Be sure to monitor your intake of nuts. Soy products, such as soy milk, tofu, edamame, and hummus, are also good carbohydrate choices.

It is very helpful to know the individual serving sizes—not to be fixated on calories but rather to be knowledgeable about food portions. The following provides a handful of examples of more popular carbohydrate foods that may assist you in constructing your nutrition periodization eating program.

Bread, Cereal, and Pasta (80 calories per serving)
- 1 slice of bread
- 2 slices of lite or reduced-calorie bread
- ½ English muffin or hamburger bun

- ¾ cup cold cereal
- ⅓ cup rice, barley, couscous, or legumes
- ½ cup pasta, bulgur, sweet potato, corn, or green peas

Vegetables (25 calories per serving)
- 1 cup raw leafy vegetables
- ½ cup other vegetables, cooked or chopped raw
- ¾ cup vegetable juice

Fruit (60 calories per serving)
- 1 small fruit (banana, apple, orange, or nectarine)
- 1 medium peach
- 1 kiwi
- ½ cup chopped, cooked, or canned fruit
- ½ cup unsweetened juice
- ½ grapefruit or mango
- 4 teaspoons jelly or jam

FIBER

The fibers of a plant form the supporting structures of the leaves, stems, and seeds. Most fiber passes through the digestive tract without providing any energy because your digestive enzymes cannot break the fibers apart. In the digestive tract, fiber can slow the absorption of nutrients, delay cholesterol absorption, bind bile for excretion, increase stool weight, and stimulate bacterial fermentation, which causes gas.

The health benefits of including fiber in your daily nutrition plan include reducing the risk of heart disease and stroke, improving the body's handling of glucose and insulin, maintaining body weight, improving the health of the digestive tract, and helping prevent constipation and hemorrhoids.

Fiber is very healthy to have within your normal eating program, but at certain times of the year—before your major competition events—it may be feasible to improve your performance by following a lower-fiber diet for a brief time. Many weight-class athletes need to reduce fiber intake significantly prior to their weigh-in so that they have less bulk in their digestive tract. Some endurance athletes have correlated GI troubles to a high-fiber eating plan prior to competition, so they also decrease their consumption. If you decide to restrict your fiber for competition reasons, it is important that you reintroduce fiber slowly and with adequate amounts of water. The "fiber taper" works on both sides. Decrease it slowly before competition and reintroduce it into your eating plan over a week to ensure that you do not experience any GI distress.

Types of Fiber

Fiber in food is classified as soluble or insoluble. Soluble fiber includes gums, mucilages, pectins, psyllium, and some hemicelluloses. Insoluble fiber includes cellulose, lignin, and some hemicelluloses. Soluble fiber gains the most attention because it functions to lower cholesterol, slow glucose absorption and transit of food, and soften stools. It is also partly fermentable into fragments that your body can use.

Table 2.5
Food Sources of Soluble Fiber

Barley and rye	Fruits and vegetables	Seeds
Legumes	Oats	Oat bran

Insoluble fiber assists with softening stools, regulating bowel movements, speeding transit of foodstuff through the small intestine, increasing fecal weight, and reducing the risk of diverticulosis, hemorrhoids, and appendicitis.

Table 2.6
Food Sources of Insoluble Fiber

Brown rice	Fruits and vegetables	Whole grains
Legumes	Seeds	Wheat bran

Table 2.7
High-Fiber Foods

Food	Portion Size	Fiber (g)
Banana	1 medium	2.4
Apple	1 medium	3.6
Orange	1 medium	2.9
Peach	1 medium	1.9
Prunes	6 medium	8.0
Carrots	½ cup	2.3
Corn	½ cup	3.6
Green peas	½ cup	3.6
Potato with skin	1 medium	2.5
Lima beans	½ cup	4.5
Navy beans	½ cup	6.0
Kidney, Pinto beans	½ cup	6.7
Bran flakes	¾ cup	4.0
Shredded wheat	1 biscuit	3.0
Air-popped popcorn	1 cup	1.0
Whole-wheat bread	1 slice	2.1
White bread	1 slice	0.4
Broccoli	½ cup	3.8
Spinach	½ cup	2.1
Zucchini	½ cup	1.6
Brown rice, cooked	½ cup	5.3
Oatmeal, dry	⅓ cup	2.8
Corn flakes	1 ounce	0.3

It is generally recommended to consume 20–35 grams of fiber each day, but, as I mentioned before, depending on your sport, weight goals, and GI challenges, you may customize your fiber intake for competitions. Table 2.7 helps you determine how to effectively get enough fiber in your diet through the foods you eat.

PROTEIN

Protein is a very important nutrient for all athletes: it provides the muscles with the amino acids they need to resynthesize and rebuild new muscle cells.

In the body, protein plays key roles in many areas, including the following:

- Enzymes: some proteins are enzymes and facilitate needed chemical reactions.
- Hormones: some hormones, which regulate body processes, are proteins, made from proteins, or require proteins in order to function.
- Antibodies: proteins form the immune system's molecules that fight disease.
- Fluid and electrolyte balance: proteins help maintain the fluid and mineral composition of various body fluids.
- Acid-base balance: proteins help maintain the acid-base balance (pH) of various body fluids by acting as buffers.
- Energy: proteins provide some of the fuel for the body's energy needs.
- Transportation: proteins help transport needed substances, such as fat, minerals, and oxygen, around the body.
- Blood clotting: proteins provide the netting on which blood clots are built.
- Structural components: proteins form integral parts of most body structures, such as skin, tendons, ligaments, membranes, muscles, organs, and bones.

Each gram of protein provides four calories. Unlike carbohydrates, after proteins are broken down into amino acids, many different things can happen to them. To understand the different fates that protein can meet in the body, it is important to first understand what makes up a protein.

A protein is comprised of amino acids. Each amino acid consists of an amine group (the nitrogen-containing part), a carbon atom with a side chain, and an acid. Each amino acid has a specific side chain that gives it its identity and chemical nature. Amino acids can be used to build new proteins or other needed compounds (such as the vitamin niacin).

If the body has a surplus of amino acids and energy, the carbon backbone of the amino acid becomes converted to fat and the nitrogen is excreted in the urine. This is why overconsuming protein is not beneficial—if you already have a good store of amino acids, the remaining protein can be stored as fat.

The protein from food that you eat travels to the stomach, where stomach acid separates the protein into shorter strands and amino acids. These then travel to the small intestine, where they are broken down further and absorbed into the blood for delivery to the cells in need of amino acids.

Types of Proteins

The two types of proteins are classified as essential and nonessential. By definition, essential proteins provide all of the amino acids that the body cannot make and thus need to obtain through food. These proteins are found in abundance in any animal product, such as meat, fish, and dairy products; soy products; and some grains, such as quinoa. Nonessential proteins provide the amino acids that your body can make. These proteins are found in foods such as legumes, seeds and nuts, grains, and vegetables.

Table 2.8
List of the Essential Amino Acids

Histidine	Isoleucine (branched-chain amino acid)	Leucine (branched-chain amino acid)
Lysine	Methionine	Phenyalanine
Threonine	Tryptophan	Valine (branched-chain amino acid)

Table 2.9
List of the Nonessential Amino Acids

Alanine	Arginine	Asparagine
Aspartic acid	Cysteine	Glutamic acid
Glutamine	Glycine	Proline
Serine	Tyrosine	

Each amino acid has different functions in your body. Table 2.10 provides you with information about each amino acid and some of the food sources in which you can find amino acids.

Table 2.10
Types, Functions, and Food Sources of Amino Acids

Amino Acid	Function	Food Sources
Histidine	A precursor to histamine that is released by the immune system during an allergic reaction. Needed for the maintenance of the myelin sheath that protects nerve cells.	Dairy, poultry, fish, meat, rye, rice, and wheat.
Isoleucine	Part of the branched-chain amino acids, which can be used as an energy source in muscle and immune cells.	Eggs, meat, poultry, fish, dairy products, oatmeal, legumes
Leucine	Part of the branched-chain amino acids, which can be used as an energy source in muscle and immune cells.	Eggs, meat, poultry, fish, dairy products, oatmeal, legumes
Lysine	Involved in the synthesis of collagen and elastin and is a precursor to carnitine.	Ground beef, Atlantic salmon, tofu, black beans, nonfat milk Whole-wheat bread, corn, spinach, egg, mozzarella cheese, peanuts
Methionine	Assists in the breakdown of fats. Can serve as an antioxidant.	Meat, fish, garlic, beans, eggs, onions, lentils, seeds, and yogurt
Phenylalanine	L-phenylalanine (the natural form) can be converted to tyrosine, which can be converted into one of several neurotransmitter molecules that have roles in brain metabolism and elevating mood and altering pain sensation.	Almonds, dairy products, avocados, peanuts, lima beans, and seeds

Table 2.10 (Continued)

Amino Acid	Function	Food Sources
Threonine	Assists in the formation of collagen and elastin.	Meat, eggs, dairy, wheat germ, beans, and nuts
Tryptophan	Tryptophan is converted in the body to 5-HTP, which can then be converted into serotonin. Serotonin can have influences on mood, sleep, and pain control.	Cottage cheese, soy protein, meat, and peanuts
Valine	Part of the branched-chain amino acids, which can be used as an energy source in muscle and immune cells.	Eggs, meat, poultry, fish, dairy products, oatmeal, legumes
Alanine	Alanine functions in the metabolism of glucose. The body can make all that it needs.	Meat, poultry, eggs, fish, dairy products, and avocado
Arginine	L-arginine (the natural and not synthetic form) is a component of the nitric oxide pathway in the body that is involved in vasodilation and cardiovascular function.	Ground beef, shredded wheat, cheddar cheese, nonfat milk, egg, brown rice, soy milk, Atlantic salmon, garbanzo beans
Asparagine	Can be hydrolyzed into aspartic acid and acts as a reservoir of amino groups in the body.	Ground beef, chicken breast, whole-wheat flour, egg, corn
Aspartic Acid	Involved in urea synthesis and can be converted into glucose and used as energy.	Ground beef, chicken breast, whole-wheat flour, egg, corn
Cysteine	A component of the antioxidant glutathione and can be converted into glucose and used as a source of energy. Can be made from methionine.	Poultry, wheat, broccoli, eggs, garlic, onions, and red peppers

(Continued)

Table 2.10 (Continued)

Amino Acid	Function	Food Sources
Glutamic Acid	An excitatory neurotransmitter and important in the metabolism of carbohydrate and fat.	Meat, poultry, fish, eggs, and dairy products
Glutamine	Serves as a precursor to synthesize other amino acids and can be made into glucose and used as energy.	Fish, meat, beans, dairy products, raw parsley, and spinach
Glycine	Required for the synthesis of DNA and the construction of RNA, bile acids, and other amino acids. Aids in the absorption of calcium.	Fish, meat, beans, and dairy products
Proline	Aids in collagen formation. Can be made from other amino acids.	Meat products
Serine	A part of brain proteins and nerve coverings and is required for the metabolism of fat, tissue growth, and immune function.	Meats, dairy products, wheat gluten, and soy products
Tyrosine	Can be synthesized from phenylalanine and is used to make epinephrine, norepinephrine, serotonin, and dopamine, which all help to regulate mood.	Meat, dairy products, eggs, almonds, avocados, and bananas

Food Sources

As mentioned previously, protein is found abundantly in many foods, including meat, dairy, and soy products, as well as nuts, grains, fruits, and vegetables. Yes, some fruits and vegetables do contain protein, although not much. Similar to the case of carbohydrates, it is easy to find foods that contain protein, even if you are a vegetarian, vegan, or do not like to eat many meat products. You may remember the days of complementary proteins, when it was said that you had to eat a nonessential protein combined with an essential protein at the same time to reap the most benefit. This is no longer the case. As long as you are eating a variety of protein food sources, your body accumulates these into an amino acid "pool" and uses amino acids as you need them. Eating any protein-containing food contributes to your amino acid pool.

Your body stores protein in its muscles. At any given time during rest, however, your body only uses approximately 2–5% of protein for energy when carbohydrates are consumed.

The following are common serving sizes for protein-rich foods:

Fat-Free and Very Low-Fat Milk and Yogurt (90 calories per serving)

- 1 cup fat-free or 1% milk
- ¾ cup plain nonfat or low-fat yogurt
- 1 cup artificially sweetened yogurt

Very Lean Protein (35 calories per serving)

- 1 ounce turkey or chicken breast (no skin)
- 1 ounce fish fillet (flounder, sole, cod, etc.), canned tuna in water, or shellfish (clams, lobster, shrimp, scallop)
- ¾ cup cottage cheese, nonfat or low-fat
- 2 egg whites
- ¼ cup egg substitute
- ½ cup cooked beans (counts as one starch also)

Lean Protein (55 calories per serving)

- 1 ounce chicken or turkey (dark meat)
- 1 ounce salmon, swordfish, or herring
- 1 ounce lean beef (roast beef, London broil, or tenderloin), veal, lamb, or pork
- 1 ounce low-fat cheese or lunch meat
- 2 medium sardines

Medium-Fat Proteins (75 calories per serving)
- 1 ounce beef, corned beef, ground beef, pork chop
- 1 whole egg
- ¼ cup ricotta cheese
- 4 ounces tofu (this is a very healthy choice)

FUELTIP

Recent research has proven that consuming protein with a carbohydrate source—rather than just a carbohydrate alone—after a workout or competition is beneficial. Several other research studies found a reduction of total free-radical buildup (by 69%), increased insulin levels (by 70%), decreased post-exercise muscle damage (by 36%), and increased muscle glycogen levels (2.2-fold). There is no doubt that the addition of protein to your nutrition plan post-workout is important and applicable. In fact, there is also good research to indicate that the addition of protein during training could aid in reducing muscle soreness and damage after exercise, which can be extremely important to strength and power athletes as well as to endurance athletes undergoing intensive or long-duration training.

The amino acid glutamine, which is found in almost every post-workout nutrition product, is also beneficial to include in your nutrition recovery protein makeup. Intense exercise decreases glutamine stores faster than the body can replenish them. When this happens, the body breaks down muscle tissue. Research has shown that glutamine supports glycogen and protein synthesis and increases nitrogen retention, making it essential for muscle repair.

Protein is an essential nutrient for athletes of all sports. The importance of timing of protein consumption and the quality of protein in relation to a workout are the determining variables that differ among athletes. I discuss that in the next chapter, as it relates to your specific training cycle and physical goals.

FUELTIP

Whey protein has become extremely popular among athletes and for good reason. It has very positive benefits to health and performance. Some athletes, however, are misinformed regarding this type of protein.

Whey protein is not a product of chemistry class, made by combining a few elements from the periodic table. It is a natural protein from dairy that is actually a by-product of cheese production. The power of whey is truly remarkable, in that it contains all of the amino acids that the body needs for regulating muscle protein synthesis, is about 95% digestible, and is rapidly absorbed in the body. To boot, it has the highest protein quality rating (followed by milk, casein, egg, soy, and beef).

The protein quality ratings get a bit technical to understand at times, but the easiest measure to focus on is the biological value (BV). This is a measurement scale that is used to determine the percentage of a nutrient that is utilized by the body. It is used frequently when comparing different protein sources and the take-home message of using BV is that it tells you how efficiently and fast your body can use the protein that you eat or drink. Whey protein isolate has the highest BV, which makes it a better "bang for your buck" protein.

Whey protein also has the highest amount of branched-chain amino acids (valine, isoleucine, and leucine), which make up about one-third of your muscle. The most important of the three is leucine. Leucine by itself has been shown to stimulate muscle protein synthesis. This means is that it can help deter muscle wasting after a tough workout. The more muscle that you can preserve, the better, from both a health and exercise perspective.

There are a few types of whey protein. Whey protein isolate is top notch: it is greater than 90% pure whey protein and contains only 1% or less of fat and lactose. It is the whey protein source that is preferred by those who experience lactose intolerance. In contrast, whey concentrate has differing levels of whey protein and contains more fat and lactose. Hands down, whey protein isolate receives the gold star for quality.

FAT

You would be hard-pressed to find foods that do not contain fat. Aside from fruits and vegetables, just about every food has some sort of fat, including snack foods such as cookies and potato chips, butter, lard, animal and dairy products, nuts, mayonnaise, shortening, soy products, salad dressings, oils, chocolate, and so on.

The fats found in foods and in your body fall into three classes. About 95% are triglycerides. The other two types are phospholipids (lecithin is one example) and sterols (cholesterol is the most well-known sterol).

On average, the body has approximately 80,000 or more calories stored as fat. Fat is essential for body processes such as body insulation, internal organ protection, nerve transmission, and, probably most important, metabolizing fat-soluble vitamins (A, D, E, and K). Although a high-fat diet can be detrimental to health, a diet that is too low in fat could potentially cause health problems also.

One gram of fat has nine calories, which is more than two times the number of calories per gram that carbohydrates or protein provide. Fat could potentially provide you with a large amount of energy if you teach your body how to use it (more on this in the last chapter, under the topic of metabolic efficiency).

The body has the ability to store much more fat than carbohydrates (see Table 2.11) because carbohydrates hold water and are quite bulky. Fat cells, on the other hand, pack tightly together with much less water and store much more energy in a smaller area. The non-healthy fats in your body can cause serious health issues, such as heart disease and high cholesterol, and having more stored fat can result in a higher body weight and fat composition, which can be detrimental to performance for some

Table 2.11
Storage Amounts of Fat in the Body

Source	Storage Form	Total Body Calories
Fat	Serum FFA	7
	Serum triglycerides	75
	Muscle triglycerides	2,500
	Adipose triglycerides	80,000

athletes. Eating the right amount and the right kinds of fat is the key to maximizing your health and performance.

The digestion of fat begins in the mouth just as it does for carbohydrates. Fat then travels to the stomach, where it separates from other compounds and floats on top. Fat does not mix with the stomach fluids, so very little digestion takes place in the stomach. From the stomach, it enters the small intestine, where it mixes with bile and pancreatic juices, which break the fat down into smaller particles. These smaller particles are then absorbed into the bloodstream.

Types of Fats

There are two classifications of fats: saturated and unsaturated. Unsaturated fats have three additional subcategories: monounsaturated, polyunsaturated, and trans fats. Saturated fats are typically solid at room temperature, like butter, and unsaturated fats are typically liquid at room temperature, like olive oil. Chemically, saturated fats have most of their fatty acids saturated with hydrogen.

Unsaturated fats have one or more fatty acids that are unsaturated. This difference in chemical structure makes a big difference when it comes to how these fats affect health.

Saturated fatty acids (SFA) often have the term "unhealthy" associated with them because they have a negative impact on heart health and could contribute to cardiovascular disease.

There has also been research linking SFA and trans fats to a higher inflammatory response in the body. Because these types of fats are not beneficial to health or performance, I recommend that no more than 5–10% of your total calories come from SFA.

The unsaturated fats, both mono- and poly-, are much better for health, because they have positive effects on heart health and can actually reduce the risk of cardiovascular disease.

Monounsaturated fatty acids (MUFA) can be found in some oils (see Table 2.12) and in foods such as avocados, olives, and nuts. Polyunsaturated fatty acids (PUFA) can be found in oils and in foods such as fish, walnuts, and flax products. MUFA should make up about 10–15% of your total daily calories, and PUFA should make up about 10% of your total daily calories.

Although trans fats are classified technically as an unsaturated fat, there is nothing healthy about them. Trans fats are polyunsaturated oils that are hardened by hydrogenation. Manufactured hydrogenated oils, in addition to being saturated, often have altered chemical shapes as well. This change in shape results in a higher risk for heart disease because trans fats can cause an increase in low-density lipoprotein (LDL), or the "bad" cholesterol, and a decrease in high-density lipoprotein (HDL), or the "good" cholesterol. Because of the chemical changes to these fats, they are worse for you than natural SFA, such as butter. Trans fats should be completely eliminated from the diet if possible.

Some food labels do not have trans fats listed on them, whereas others do. Thus it is important to look at the ingredients list for the term "partially hydrogenated oils." If it states this on the label, you know a product contains trans fats. Stay away from these products or significantly limit the amount that you eat. Almost all processed foods and snacks have trans fat in them, so beware and read the ingredients list first. Additionally, some energy bars will have trans fats due to their chocolate coating. The body can synthesize saturated and monounsaturated fats, but not all of the polyunsaturated fats that make them essential to health and performance.

Table 2.12
Fat Composition of Common Oils

Oil Comparisons 1 tablespoon	SFA	MUFA	PUFA	Omega 6	Omega 3
Olive	2	10	1	1	0
Canola	1	9	4	3	1
Coconut	12	<1	<1	0	0
Corn	2	4	7	7	0
Flaxseed	1	3	9	2	7
Grapeseed	1	2	10	9	0
Palm kernal	11	1.5	<1	0	0
Peanut	2	6	4	4	0
Safflower	1	2	10	10	0
Sunflower	1	11	1	1	0
Sesame	2	5	6	6	0
Wheat germ	3	2	8	7	1

*Source: USDA Nutrient Database

Essential Fatty Acids

Omega-6 and omega-3 fatty acids are essential polyunsaturated fatty acids, or essential fatty acids (EFA), which cannot be made by the body's cells. The cells cannot convert one fat to another. Therefore these fats must be provided by the food you eat.

Essential fatty acids have many very important health functions including the following:

- Regulating blood pressure
- Forming blood clots
- Regulating blood lipids
- Acting like hormones
- Assisting the immune response
- Decreasing the inflammation response to injury and infection

Additionally, EFAs serve as structural parts of cell membranes, constitute a major part of the lipids of the brain and nerves, and are essential to normal growth and vision in infants and children. A common misconception among athletes, however, is that polyunsaturated fats are created equal. In fact, the exact opposite is true, and it is important to know the differences in the two main types of polyunsaturated fats, as it could have a profound effect on not only your health, but also your performance. The main difference lies in the metabolism of both of these polyunsaturated fats. In the metabolism of these fats, both compete for one particular shared enzyme in order to be metabolized. This can be somewhat problematic because omega-6 fats predominate in most eating programs for athletes, and because of this, these fats take preference of the shared enzymes and are preferentially metabolized instead of omega-3 fats. This leads to a metabolic dominance of omega-6 fats, which can have a negative impact on health and performance in terms of the inflammation response (more on this in the last chapter under the topic inflammation).

FUELTIP

You may have heard of the terms EPA and DHA before. These are fatty acids that are beneficial to both your health and performance. There are very few food sources of these fats (see Table 2.13), however, so many athletes reach to fish oil supplements. Taking supplements and including a good amount of these fats through different food sources is extremely beneficial.

Table 2.13
Common Food Sources of Omega-6 and Omega-3 Fats

Food Source	Serving Size	Omega-6:3 ratio
Salmon	3 ounces (wild)	1:1.5
Ground flax	1 tablespoon	1:3
Trout	3 ounces (rainbow, wild)	2:1
Walnuts	1 cup	4.5:1
Halibut	3 ounces	1:2
Sardines	1 ounce (in tomato sauce)	1:2
Tuna fish	3 ounces (canned in water)	1:1

The goal for you would be to decrease the omega-6 to omega-3 ratio so that you eat more omega-3 fats, which would then lead to a better metabolic conversion to the beneficial compounds EPA and DHA.

Serving Sizes

The following serving sizes will provide the information regarding different sources of fat.

Fat (45 calories per serving)

- 1 teaspoon oil, butter, stick margarine, or mayonnaise
- 1 tablespoon reduced-fat margarine or mayonnaise, salad dressing, or cream cheese
- 2 tablespoons lite cream cheese
- ⅛ avocado
- 8 large black olives
- 10 large stuffed green olives
- 1 slice bacon

Another form of fat that has become very popular among athletes is medium chain triglycerides, commonly referred to as MCTs. MCTs are made from coconut oil. The oil is split into glycerol and long-chain and medium-chain fatty acids. The medium chains are then rejoined with glycerol to form MCTs. This is important because semi-synthetic MCTs have different characteristics from other fat that you eat. Specifically, MCTs mix easily with liquid and have a smaller molecular size than ordinary fat, which allows them to be absorbed more rapidly into the intestine. They are also transported differently and are not dependent on the carnitine system for transport across the mitochondrial membrane. Because carnitine transport is thought to be one of the factors that slows down the oxidation of fat, it is believed that MCTs will be oxidized faster, which means that you will obtain energy quicker.

Do they actually work, is the real question. Research has discovered that MCTs are rapidly emptied from the stomach and available for use as fuel during exercise, and it is better to take them in combination with carbohydrate, which will not inhibit glycogen utilization. Keep in mind that consuming 30 grams of MCTs seems to be the most that athletes can tolerate. More than this can lead to stomach cramps and diarrhea.

Carbohydrates are still vitally important in training but the MCT story is intriguing. Because MCT use is limited by the amount that can be tolerated without causing GI distress, it has been found that it can only contribute between 3–7% of the total energy expenditure during some types of exercise. Whether or not this can function as a significant improvement in performance is still under debate.

Water

Of the six nutrients essential to life, water is by far the most important. Water makes up about 60–75% of total body weight. Drinking too little water or losing too much through sweating can inhibit your ability to exercise and perform at an optimal level.

Water keeps the body hydrated, acts in the blood as a transport mechanism, eliminates metabolic waste products in urine, dissipates heat through sweat, helps to digest food, lubricates joints, and cushions organs. Water is an essential nutrient that is crucial to survival as well as athletic performance.

Fluid needs of athletes differ greatly and the general public guidelines do not apply to athletes. I will explain some fairly easy techniques to assess hydration status so you ensure that you are staying well hydrated throughout the day, but first let me explain the physiological drive to drink.

Thirst, defined as a conscious awareness of the desire for water and other fluids, usually controls water intake. The physiological drive to drink is controlled by three factors: a decrease in blood volume, an increase in blood osmolarity (the total concentration of particles in solute), and a decrease in the flow of saliva. These markers will ultimately lead to sending a signal to your brain, which will increase thirst and make you drink more fluid.

FUELTIP

The truth of the matter is that most athletes will enter a training session dehydrated most of the time. If you work out first thing in the morning, you will be in a dehydrated state as a result of sleeping, no matter how much you try to drink beforehand. I recommend athletes try not to schedule quality (defined as high intensity and/or long duration) workouts early in the day if they can control it. These types of workouts are much better suited for later in the day, once you have had a chance to eat and drink. Of course, this does assume that you hydrate properly throughout the day.

Thirst can also be blunted by exercise or overridden by the mind. Your body will usually only signal you to replace two-thirds of your sweat losses. Being one-third behind in fluid consumption can be significant, especially if you have multiple training sessions in one day.

There are a few methods of monitoring hydration status, some easier and more practical than others. The first method is through observing the color of your urine. Although not 100% accurate, it will provide you with a start to monitoring your hydration status. With the exception of your morning "pit stop," your urine should be no darker than the color of straw (pale yellow). If it resembles the color of apple juice, then you know you have not been doing a good job at consuming fluids. If it is bright yellow, you may be taking in an overabundance of B vitamins.

The second somewhat simple method of monitoring your daily hydration status is by the frequency of your pit stops. Realistically, if you urinate every 2–3 hours, it is a good marker that you are maintaining fluid balance and hydrating well. If you urinate more frequently, you may be drinking too many caffeinated beverages or too much plain water (water, when consumed alone, is excreted quite efficiently by the kidneys).

FUELTIP

To stay hydrated throughout the day, carry a water bottle or closed container of water with you wherever you go. I have noticed that athletes are less likely to drink often if they choose an open cup or glass because it is not portable. Some athletes have great success in consuming more water when they carry a gallon jug of water with them, while others have more success when they carry a smaller 16–20 ounce bottle. It does not matter which you choose as long as you drink from it. Remember, as water gets warm, you may not want to drink it, so be sure that whatever size container you choose, you finish its content before it becomes unpalatable.

It is also a good strategy to keep a container at work, one in the car, and a few ready in the refrigerator so that they are easy to grab anytime. The more accessible they are, the more successful you will be at staying hydrated during the day.

Fear not if you are an athlete who just doesn't like drinking water. Another great way to meet your daily fluid needs is by eating the right foods. Certain foods, such as fruits and vegetables, have large water content. Your fluid needs do not need to be met by water alone. You can also stay hydrated with other beverages such as iced tea or lemonade, and in case you are wondering, it has been found that the caffeine in some of these drinks is not as dehydrating as once thought. Just be sure to balance your consumption of the caffeinated beverages with their noncaffeinated counterparts throughout the day.

The last easy-to-implement method of tracking your fluid intake is by using a simple bathroom scale. Although I am not a fan of using scales in general, they are very applicable in fluid balance testing and ensuring that your daily hydration plan is sound. The following chart will help guide you, should you choose to use a scale to monitor your hydration status.

Hydration Status	% Body Weight Change
Well hydrated	+1 to −1
Minimal dehydration	−1 to −3
Significant dehydration	−4 to −5
Serious dehydration	More than 5

Vitamins

Vitamins are metabolic catalysts that regulate biochemical reactions within the body. To date, 13 vitamins have been discovered, each with a specific function. Interestingly, there is no scientific research that proves that extra vitamins offer a competitive edge. Obviously, if you have a vitamin deficiency, a vitamin supplement can help to correct that; however, vitamin deficiencies are usually related to a larger medical problem that needs attention and are somewhat rare for athletes who consume the proper quantity of food. For some weight cutting and aesthetic sports where calories are restricted, however, vitamin deficiencies do occur. Keeping this in mind, some vitamins are stored in the body in large amounts (vitamins A, D, E, and K), while others are stored in smaller amounts (vitamins B and C), so it is virtually impossible for a nutritional deficiency to occur overnight.

Vitamins are catalysts that are needed for metabolic processes and they do not provide direct energy. There are some athletes who may be at higher risk for nutritional deficiencies and should consider taking a daily multi-vitamin. These at-risk athletes include:

- Athletes who eat less than 1200–1500 calories per day
- Athletes who are allergic to certain foods
- Athletes who are lactose intolerant, leading to low amounts of riboflavin and calcium
- Athletes who are pregnant
- Athletes who are contemplating pregnancy; folic acid, iron, and calcium are important during conception and pregnancy

- Athletes who are complete vegetarians; vegetarianism could result in low amounts of vitamins B_{12} and D, riboflavin, iron, and zinc

The bottom line is that as an athlete, it is a good idea to try to get your vitamins from foods first. I have worked with many athletes, however, who cannot physically eat enough food in a day to remain in energy balance; thus their vitamin and mineral needs may be justified by taking a daily multi-vitamin.

Standards for Micronutrient Intake

The Institute of Medicine established standards of various nutrient intakes, termed Dietary Reference Intakes (DRIs), and are based on the assessment of the estimated average requirement (EAR), the recommended dietary allowances (RDA), the adequate intake (AI), and the tolerable upper intake level (UL). This system replaced the old nomenclature of the RDA, and although this alphabet soup can become a bit confusing, the main intent of the DRI is to lower the risk of developing chronic disease through balanced nutrient intake. For athletes, the DRI may not meet the demands of a high level of training for some vitamins and minerals, but using the range of DRI to UL based on training cycle and load should provide more than enough nutrients to sustain a high level of training and competition. I would strongly recommend not using the "more is better" approach when consuming vitamins and minerals in excess of the UL.

DIETARY REFERENCE INTAKES DEFINITIONS

Estimated Average Requirement (EAR)

- A daily nutrient intake value that is estimated to meet the requirement of half of the healthy individuals in a life stage and gender group. This is used to assess dietary adequacy and is the basis for the RDA.

Recommended Dietary Allowance (RDA)

- The average daily dietary intake level that is sufficient to meet the nutrient requirements of nearly all healthy individuals in a particular life stage and gender group.

Adequate Intake (AI)

- A recommended intake value based on observed or experimentally determined approximations or estimates, assumed to be adequate, of nutrient intake by a group or groups of healthy individuals. This is used when an RDA cannot be determined.

Tolerable Upper Intake Level (UL)

- The highest level of daily nutrient intake that is likely to pose no risk of adverse health effects for almost all individuals in the general population.

Below is an overview of the different vitamins, their functions, food sources, recommended intakes, signs/symptoms of toxicity, and deficiency of each. The food sources column represents the more common sources of the vitamins; it is not a comprehensive list of sources. In addition, the DRI values are for adults who are not pregnant, lactating, injured, or not between the ages of 19–70 years old.

Water Soluble Vitamins	Function	Food Sources	DRI/day	UL/day	Toxicity	Deficiency
B$_1$ (thiamin)	Helps metabolism of carbohydrate into energy	Potatoes, fish, bananas, ham, chicken, bread, cereal, and enriched rice	Females: 1.1 mg Males: 1.2 mg	UL not established	None known	Heart disease, confusion, anorexia, calf pain, weakness

(Continued)

Water Soluble Vitamins	Function	Food Sources	DRI/day	UL/day	Toxicity	Deficiency
B₂ (riboflavin)	Necessary for energy release and for healthy skin, mucous membranes, and nervous system	Spinach, steak, cottage cheese, milk, oranges, apples, and enriched bread and cereal	Females: 1.1 mg Males: 1.3 mg	UL not established	None known	Fatigue; weakness; cracked and dry skin at corners of mouth, nose, and eyes; bright light sensitivity; inflamed tongue
B₃ (niacin)	Helps metabolism of food into energy, necessary for growth and production of hormones	Tuna, potatoes, halibut, peas, cereal, corn, mushrooms, peanut butter, ground beef, and enriched bread	Females: 14 mg Males: 16 mg	Females and males: 35 mg	Hepatitis and gastric ulcers; flushing, tingling, and burning sensations of extremities	Weakness, lethargy, anorexia, dementia, skin rash
B₆	Necessary for synthesis and breakdown of amino acids, aids in metabolism of carbohydrates	Peanut butter, chick peas, chicken, spinach, cereal, potatoes, bananas, and lima beans	Females: 1.3–1.5 mg Males: 1.3–1.7 mg	Females and males: 100 mg	Loss of sensation in the limbs, loss of balance and coordination	Muscle weakness, depression, nausea, depressed immune system, mouth sores, convulsions
Folic Acid	Necessary for production of blood cells and a healthy nervous system	Spinach, broccoli, green beans, peas, lentils, asparagus,	Females and males: 400 mcg	Females and males: 1000 mcg	None known	Neural tube defects, megaloblastic anemia

(Continued)

Water Soluble Vitamins	Function	Food Sources	DRI/day	UL/day	Toxicity	Deficiency
		mushrooms, lima beans, and oranges				
Biotin	Necessary for metabolism of carbohydrates, protein, and fat	Nuts, split peas, eggs, cauliflower, and mushrooms	Females and males: 30 mcg	UL not established	Unknown	Rare but can include depression, dermatitis, anorexia, muscle pain
Pantothenic Acid	Necessary for metabolism of carbohydrates, protein, and fat	Eggs, peanuts, mixed vegetables, steak, fish, wheat germ, and broccoli	Females and males: 5 mg	UL not established	Unknown	Unknown
B$_{12}$	Necessary for the synthesis of red and white blood cells, aids in metabolism of food	Chicken, meat, eggs, milk, and yogurt	Females and males: 2.4 mcg	UL not established	Unknown	Pernicious anemia, weakness
C	Necessary for healthy connective tissue, bones, teeth, and cartilage, supports a healthy immune system	Bell peppers, broccoli, strawberries, oranges, potatoes, tomatoes, and kiwi	Females: 75 mg Males: 90 mg	Females and males: 2,000 mg	Increased risk of kidney stones	Rare but can include deterioration of muscles and tendons, bleeding gums (scurvy)

(Continued)

Water Soluble Vitamins	Function	Food Sources	DRI/day	UL/day	Toxicity	Deficiency
A (retinol)	Necessary for healthy eyes, skin, and the linings of the digestive, urinary tract, and the nose	Milk, dried apricots, squash, carrots, spinach, and fortified food products	Females: 700 mcg Males: 900 mcg	Females and males: 3,000 mcg	Liver damage, bone malformations	Headache, vomiting, night blindness, dry skin, irritability, increased risk of infection
D	Necessary for calcium and phosphorus metabolism and for healthy bones and teeth	Milk, fortified foods such as cereal; sunlight is also a good source of non-food vitamin D	Females and males: 5 mcg	Females and males: 50 mcg	Nausea, loss of muscle function, diarrhea, organ damage	Osteomalacia, increased risk of stress fractures and osteoporosis
E	Necessary for nourishing and strengthening cells, functions as an antioxidant	Wheat germ, sunflower seeds, almonds, and whole-wheat grains	Females and males: 15 mg	Females and males: 1000 mg	Unknown	Rare
K	Necessary for blood clotting	Cabbage, spinach, broccoli, and kale	Females: 90 mcg Males: 120 mcg	UL not established	Unknown	Rare

The following chart is a summary of important body functions related to each vitamin.

Vitamin	Cofactors and activators for energy metabolism	Nervous system function and muscle contraction	Hemoglobin synthesis	Immune function	Antioxidant function	Bone metabolism
Thiamin	X	X				
Riboflavin	X	X				
B$_6$	X	X	X	X		
Folic acid		X	X			
B$_{12}$		X	X			
Niacin	X	X				
Pantothenic acid	X					
Biotin	X					
C				X	X	
A				X	X	
D						X
K						X
E				X	X	

Vitamins are extremely important for sustaining optimal health and can play a significant role in athletic performance. It is recommended to begin with a solid food foundation to acquire the vitamins that your body needs before choosing a supplement.

Minerals

Minerals are elements that combine in various ways to form structures of the body and regulate body processes. Minerals are found in abundance in most foods that you eat, but they do not serve as a source of energy. The minerals magnesium, sodium, calcium, potassium, zinc, and iron are the most popular among athletes because of their impact on hydration and cramping, oxygen delivery, and the health of the immune system.

Below is an overview of the different minerals, their functions, food sources, recommended intakes, signs/symptoms of toxicity, and deficiency of each. The food sources column represents a more common source of minerals; it is not a comprehensive list of mineral sources. In addition, the DRI values are for adults who are not pregnant, lactating, injured, or not between the ages of 19–50 years old.

Mineral (macro)	Function	Food Sources	DRI/day	UL/day	Toxicity	Deficiency
Calcium	Necessary for bone formation, enzyme reactions, and muscle contractions	Dairy products, green leafy vegetables, and beans	Females and males: 1,000 mg	Females and males: 2,500 mg	Constipation; malabsorption of iron, magnesium and zinc; cardiac arrhythmia; kidney stones	Poor muscle function, osteoporosis
Phosphorus	Necessary for building bones and teeth, aids in metabolism	Meat, fish, dairy products, and carbonated beverages	Females and males: 700 mg	Females and males: 4,000 mg	Rare but can include GI distress and low bone density	Rare but can include muscle weakness and low bone density
Magnesium	Necessary for energy production, muscle relaxation, and nerve signal conduction	Whole grains, nuts, meats, and beans	Females: 320 mg Males: 420 mg	Females and males: 350 mg (if taken as supplements)	Vomiting, diarrhea, nausea	Rare but can include muscle cramps, cardiac arrythmias, muscle weakness
Sodium	Necessary for nerve impulses, muscle action, and body fluid balance	Table salt and most foods, except fruits	Females and males: 1,500 mg	Females and males: 2,300 mg (some athletes may require much more than the UL)	Hypertension (in a small percentage)	Hyponatremia, muscle cramping, vomiting; nausea, seizures, coma, anorexia

(Continued)

Mineral (macro)	Function	Food Sources	DRI/day	UL/day	Toxicity	Deficiency
Potassium	Necessary for fluid balance, muscle action, and glycogen and protein synthesis	Bananas, orange juice, fruits, and vegetables	Females and males: 4,700 mg	UL not established	Hyperkalemia (may lead to cardiac arrythmias and altered heart function)	Hypokalemia (associated with anorexia, muscle cramping, and arrythmias)
Chloride	Necessary for stomach acid production, nerve function, water balance	Table salt	Females and males: 2,000–2,300 mg	Females and males: 3,600 mg	Hypertension (in a small percentage)	Vomiting, convulsions (rare)
Selenium	Functions as an antioxidant	Meat, seafood, and whole grains	Females and males: 55 mcg	Females and males: 400 mcg	Rare but can include hair loss, GI distress, and nausea	Rare but can include heart damage
Chromium	Necessary for glucose uptake	Whole grains, meat, and cheese	Females: 25 mcg Males: 35 mcg	UL not established	Not likely	Glucose intolerance
Manganese	Necessary for bone and tissue development and fat synthesis	Nuts, whole grains, beans, tea, fruits, and vegetables	Females: 1.8 mg Males: 2.3 mg	Females and males: 11 mg	Fatigue, confusion, neurological issues	Poor growth and development in children
Iodine	Necessary for regulating metabolism	Iodized salt and seafood	Females and males: 150 mcg	Females and males: 1,100 mcg	Inadequate production of thyroxine	Enlarged thyroid gland (goiter), obesity

(Continued)

Mineral (macro)	Function	Food Sources	DRI/day	UL/day	Toxicity	Deficiency
Zinc	Necessary for tissue growth and healing, immune health, and gonadal development	Meat, shellfish, oysters, and whole grains	Females: 8 mg Males: 11 mg	Females and males: 40 mg	Impaired immune system, nausea, slow wound healing	Impaired immune function and wound healing, dry skin, anorexia
Copper	Necessary for hemoglobin formation, energy production, and immune health	Whole grains, beans, nuts, dried fruit, and shellfish	Females and males: 900 mcg	Females and males: 10,000 mcg	Rare but can include nausea and vomiting	Rare but can include anemia
Iron	Necessary for hemoglobin formation, muscle growth and function, and energy production	Meat, beans, dried fruit, some green, leafy vegetables	Females: 18 mg Males: 8 mg	Females and males: 45 mg	Hemochromatosis, liver damage	Fatigue, low energy metabolism, lower resistance to infection

The following chart is a summary of important body functions related to each mineral.

Mineral	Cofactors and activators for energy metabolism	Nervous system function and muscle contraction	Hemoglobin synthesis	Immune function	Antioxidant function	Bone metabolism
Sodium		X				
Potassium		X				
Calcium		X				X
Magnesium	X	X		X		X

Mineral	Cofactors and activators for energy metabolism	Nervous system function and muscle contraction	Hemoglobin synthesis	Immune function	Antioxidant function	Bone metabolism
Iron	X		X		X	
Zinc	X			X	X	
Copper	X				X	
Chromium	X					
Phosphorus	X					X
Iodine	X					
Chloride		X				
Manganese	X					X
Selenium					X	

Both vitamins and minerals also contain antioxidants, which are extremely important to all athletes. Refer to the Supplements chapter for more in-depth information about these highly beneficial substances.

SUMMARY

Your nutritional needs will differ based on your sport, position, weight goals, and training cycle. I do not like to provide general guidelines such as percentages of total calories or ranges, as I believe they do not provide accurate information for a successful performance nutrition plan.

3

Nutrition Periodization

It is typical for many athletes to concern themselves with their nutrition a few days to a week before competitions. This "old school" method of using nutrition does not maximize performance gains during competition. As you learned in the first chapter, the concept of physical periodization is to provide the proper training methods and properly timed training load for you to attain your goals. However, the best constructed training plan is not useful unless you first consider the impact of other extrinsic factors that affect physical training and recovery.

Nutrition certainly tops this list as one of the most important limiters to training. It is certainly no secret that improper fueling or hydrating can stop a training session short, significantly slow an athlete down, or, in more serious instances, create an unplanned trip to the hospital. Nutrition is more than simply knowing what a carbohydrate, protein, or fat is. The future of nutrition involves periodizing your eating plan to support your physical training plan. My mantra, "eat to train, don't train to eat," is the key to knowing what and when to eat as well as why to eat. This chapter certainly challenges you to think outside of the box, but once you are able to understand and implement the nutrition periodization principles fully, you will be on your way to a higher level of performance.

THE IMPORTANT ROLE OF NUTRITION

Some athletes use a balance of quantitative and qualitative methods to provide a systematic approach to their training and competitions. Methodical planning strategies are used with a great deal of science and technology, but what continues to surprise me is that some athletes do not spend as much time planning their nutrition program as they do their training program. I am certainly not promoting an obsessive-compulsive behavior in planning every meal and keeping track of every calorie consumed throughout the day. I am promoting the simple fact that nutrition must be taken a bit more seriously in order to support the different energy expenditures seen year-round. If you know that you are entering a high-volume and low-intensity training cycle, eat to support this. Likewise, if the intensity is about to be turned up and your volume drops, your nutrition should change. Each time your physical training program changes, your nutrition should be changing to support these different energy needs.

Maintaining proper nutrition throughout the year does not, in itself, make you stronger or faster. However, nutrition supports your body and provides the nutrients needed to improve your health, strength, speed, power, and endurance while helping maintain a healthy immune system, body weight, and body composition.

Throughout my career, working with all types, ages, and abilities of athletes, I have learned that changing either body weight or body composition resides at the top of the goal list. You will learn more about this in much detail in Chapter 4, but let me simply reinforce that the manipulation of aesthetic appearance, whether for looks or optimal performance, is the main reason for the birth of the nutrition periodization concept. If you think about it, it is fairly easy to figure out the quantity and quality of foods and drinks to consume before, during, and after training. Pick up any good sports nutrition book or visit any reputable sports nutrition Web site, and you find these guidelines. The challenge lies in the planning and implementation of these factors in order to influence body weight and composition positively at the right time of the year to elicit the greatest benefits for optimal performance. If you can treat nutrition with all the care that you give your physical training, you will certainly reap more health and performance benefits than you will by simply waiting until a day or two before your big competition.

As you will learn in this chapter, there are certain times of the year during your physical periodization cycles when your nutrition must change to supply the right mix of nutrients to support an improvement in performance. There are other times of the year when your nutrition should be cycled to have a positive influence on your body weight and composition in order to propel your body to a higher level of performance.

Don't let nutrition take a back seat to your training. Your eating program supports your body so that you are able to train, not the other way around. It is the missing link that you need to feel better before, during, and after your competitions. Do not underestimate the power of periodizing your nutrition to support your training. If you neglect your nutrition, it will come back and bite you!

The concepts of nutrition periodization are not complex. In fact, as I state throughout this book, "simple is sustainable." The simpler the concept is, the simpler the execution is and the easier it is for athletes to adopt the principles fully throughout their training cycles. The five components of the nutrition periodization model include the following:

1. Manipulate body weight
2. Manipulate body composition
3. Improve metabolic efficiency
4. Promote a healthy immune system
5. Support physical periodization

Along with the concepts are the goals of nutrition periodization (remember, simple is sustainable):

1. To enhance health
2. To improve performance
3. To manipulate body weight and composition

FUELTIP

Of course, there will be athletes who don't truly grasp the concept of nutrition periodization or who think that nutrition cannot affect their athleticism because they are already great athletes. I worked with a Division I college football linebacker, and we had many conversations about why eating fast food every day for two meals would not help his performance on the field. I knew it was a lost battle, but I kept at him, explaining to him the benefits of putting the right "fuel" in his body. He was a great athlete, with great genetics, and he required high-octane fuel, not economy-grade fuel. However, he was wired from a very young age to eat this way and had continued his comfortable habits into college. I knew I would not change him over the season, but my goal was to replace one of his fast food meals with one from a campus dining hall. Would it affect his performance in the short term? Probably not. He was an exceptional athlete. But I was concerned about his long-term goal to play in the National Football League (NFL). If I could begin to make a slight change now, he might be more successful if he reached his goal of playing professionally. This is a great example of small changes that can be implemented and that can have tremendous gains in the future.

He eventually gave up one fast food meal per day, went on to have a great season, and was drafted the following year. Is there a correlation that can be drawn? Who knows? But by simply educating him enough as to the value of high-octane foods and proper timing, I hope that he enjoys an illustrious professional football career. Even though it may not sound like a huge success, the seed was planted, and I believe that it will continue to grow as he waters it throughout his career.

When I began writing the first edition of this book, I could honestly state that 95% of the athletes with whom I have worked wanted to change the way they look (i.e., manipulation of body weight and composition). Since then, having worked with hundreds of additional athletes in many different sports, I have increased this number to 100%. It is extremely rare for me to find the athlete who does not have the goal of losing body fat, weight, or improving lean muscle mass. These are the most common themes I have seen in all my years as a sport dietitian.

I mentioned the concepts and goals of nutrition periodization, but the last piece of the puzzle of the nutrition periodization concept is the application principles, including the following:

1. Planning
2. Developing
3. Implementing
4. Quantity of food
5. Quality of food
6. Timing of food

Of these six principles, which do you think poses the most challenge to an athlete? I ask this question to every group with whom I interact, and, surprisingly, most of the answers I receive are the quantity, quality, and timing of food. Although these may appear to be the most troublesome components, they are actually the simplest. The most difficult are the planning, developing, and implementing in which qualitative and psychological factors have a greater influence than quantitative factors. There is a more emotional connection in planning, developing, and implementing an eating plan than in simply drinking 20 ounces of a sports drink a few hours before a workout. Are you beginning to see the difference?

Once the psyche becomes involved in planning or implementing anything that involves food, an emotional attachment to the food is formed. It is human nature and, quite honestly, it is often the limiting factor in any athlete's quest for better eating. As you learn how to control your mind and use it to its fullest potential, you become better at controlling the planning, development, and implementation process of foods. Eventually, you become more independent and self-sustainable with your eating program. If you can control your mind, you control your body!

PERIODIZATION AND NUTRITION PLANNING

Athletes follow specific periodization cycles throughout their year, some of which I mentioned in the previous chapter. No matter what name is given to the periodization or the progression, one thing always remains constant: volume and intensity (the training load) increase and decrease throughout an athlete's training year. With these changes come corresponding increases or decreases of stress on the body, which leads to different nutrient needs at different times. Athletes who are not nutritionally prepared before a quality training session do not receive the same positive physiological training adaptations as athletes who are prepared and who place their nutrition on the top of their priority list.

Nutrition periodization does not need to be complicated. The basic premise is that as long as you alter your eating patterns to match your training needs and energy expenditure based on your body weight and composition goals, you will be successful. However, it has been my experience many times when talking with athletes that, even though body weight/composition goals may be known, training cycles may be the unknown variable. If you have a coach, sit down with him/her and discuss your annual training plan. If you know when your competitions are, you can better adjust your nutrition. If you are self-coached, you do not have to have a complex plan. Rather, simply identify your key competitions and work backward to determine the best time to manipulate your body weight/composition that will not have a negative impact on performance.

ATHLETE DIFFERENCES

Athletes are different, but there are some similarities in energy systems that are shared among sports. I group the sports by categories: team/individual (soccer, football, basketball, golf, track and field), weight-class/aesthetic (boxing, wrestling, weightlifting, figure skating, gymnastics, synchronized swimming), and endurance (triathlon, swimming, long-distance and cross-country running, cycling, rowing, canoe, and kayak).

Because of individual differences inter- and intra-sport, macronutrient intake varies greatly. Although it is tempting to classify the lower ranges of the macronutrients for lower training levels and weight loss, this is not always the case, as I describe in each of the mesocycle nutrition goals. The ranges provide a starting point for you, a foundation of knowledge to begin adapting your eating program to your training program. As I previously mentioned, your training load changes largely dictate when and how you shift the quality and quantity of the calories that you eat. Sports nutrition for athletes of all ages, abilities, and types has a strong science background, but when it comes to applying it to your specific needs, it becomes more of an art. I provide you with the quantitative numbers that science has given us, but I also use my art, through working with different sports and athletes, to apply these nutrient ranges to the different training cycles.

The macronutrient ranges for athletes that have been cited in scientific research include 3–19 grams of carbohydrate per kilogram of body weight, 1.2–2.5 grams of protein per kilogram of body weight, and 0.8–3.0 grams of fat per kilogram of body weight. The ranges are large because of the many differences among athletes, their body weight/composition changes, and their competition cycle(s). Each sport differs based on the distance (sprint distance to Ironman distance triathlon, 100-meter sprinter to marathon runner), the position (football wide receiver versus offensive lineman), and the body weight classes in some sports such as weightlifting, wrestling, and boxing. Because of these differences, which macronutrient range an athlete should follow cannot be generalized based purely on sport and/or position. Because so much of nutrition periodization focuses on body weight/composition manipulation, athletes often fluctuate within these ranges throughout their training year(s). I classify each training cycle in this chapter with the associated macronutrient ranges that make sense for most athletes to follow.

There is fantastic scientific research being conducted in the field of sports nutrition. For example, during the first writing of this book, it was shown that the human body could absorb about 1 gram of carbohydrate per minute of moderately intense exercise. Just recently it has been shown that the body can absorb upward of 1.75 grams of carbohydrate per minute if fed a high amount of carbohydrate (2.4 grams per minute). Based on the primary author's recommendations, it is more realistic at this time to consume 1–1.5 grams of carbohydrate per minute to ensure adequate GI emptying without incurring GI distress. The guidelines that follow should always be tried in training under competition simulation training, that is, at the same intensity at which you will be competing.

The research is beneficial; however, the real-life application of these findings may not be the easiest to implement. Athletes in water sports, such as swimming, sailing, canoe/kayak, and rowing, often do not have the luxury of following a set nutrition plan because much of their fueling regimens depend on rest breaks, which sometimes cannot be planned. Players of team sports, such as football, baseball, soccer, and basketball, are also confined to period/inning changes or a halftime. Those engaged in weight and aesthetic class sports, such as wrestling, gymnastics, figure skating, and boxing, may have more frequent opportunities for nourishment, but because of the nature of the sports, water is often used instead of calorie-containing products.

As you can see, the research states that athletes can absorb more carbohydrates, but this may not be applicable for some athletes. Understanding each sport's needs is crucial to being able to recommend the proper quantities of carbohydrate, protein, and fat.

As I mentioned before, nutrition periodization is not meant to be complicated or difficult. It is meant to help you achieve peak health and performance by encouraging you to make slight changes in your nutrition during each of your physical periodization cycles. To help you make these changes, I use the same physical periodization cycles that were discussed in Chapter 1 and apply the specific nutrition periodization principles to each cycle so that it is easy for you to combine nutrition with your training program.

Nutrition Periodization

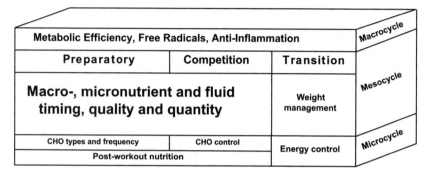

Figure 3.1 Nutrition Periodization

Figure 3.1 describes the concept of nutrition periodization in graphic form. You can see that there are specific macrocycle, mesocycle, and microcycle nutrition goals, depending upon which training cycle you are in throughout the year.

MACROCYCLE NUTRITION GUIDELINES

There are a handful of nutrition guidelines that apply year-round regardless of what type of athlete you are or what training cycle you may be in at any given time. These guidelines have the primary goal of improving health, with performance as a secondary goal. In the following, you will find specific nutrient needs and timing recommendations with notes that provide more background and possible implementation strategies.

Oxidative Stress

A first important step in macrocycle eating is to reduce the amount of cellular oxidative stress that your body experiences. This oxidative stress, referred to as reactive oxygen species, is more commonly known to athletes as free radicals. Free radicals are atoms with unpaired electrons that can be formed when oxygen interacts with certain molecules. These highly reactive free radicals can then impart damage to the cell membrane and DNA. Once this happens, the cellular functioning can decrease, which can affect many body processes. Enter the nutrition solution—antioxidants. The body has internal enzyme systems that help scavenge these free radicals, but the body can be overloaded at certain times, such as with strenuous exercise, being at a high altitude, or in a polluted environment, and under stress.

Antioxidants, acting as scavengers, interact with free radicals and can stop the damaging chain reaction of cellular damage. Choosing foods rich in beta-carotene, vitamin C, vitamin E, selenium, and zinc can help support immune function and quench free radical production.

FUELTIP

Eating foods that are rich in phytochemicals—plant compounds that have a positive effect on health and help in many disease states—and antioxidants helps keep your immune system strong as your training load fluctuates throughout the year.

Good sources of beta-carotene are carrots and sweet potatoes. Good sources of vitamin C are oranges, kiwis, strawberries, and grapefruit. Vitamin E can be found in nuts and green leafy vegetables. Zinc can be found in oysters, red meat, poultry, beans, nuts, whole grains, and dairy products. Food sources of selenium include brazil nuts, tuna, and beef.

Beneficial Fats

Focusing your attention on including more polyunsaturated and monounsaturated fats and less saturated and trans fats can help improve your health significantly. These fats have different responses in the body in terms of blood lipids, and they can influence total cholesterol, triglycerides, low-density lipoproteins (bad cholesterol), and high-density lipoproteins (healthy cholesterol).

FUELTIP

A good rule of thumb is to limit your saturated fat intake to 10% or less of total calories, or 1 gram or less of saturated fat for every 100 calories eaten. This is very easy to do by checking the nutrition facts label for saturated fat and comparing it to the total calories per serving. These fats are found mostly in animal products, processed foods such as cakes, cookies, and chips, and energy bars that have a chocolate or other type of coating. Be sure to read the label closely.

Trans fats are even worse for your health than saturated fats. You should completely eliminate these from your diet if at all possible. Looking at the nutrition facts label for the quantity of trans fat in a product may not be enough. If a product contains less than 0.49 grams of trans fat per serving, the manufacturer can list the trans fat value as zero on the label. To be a smart consumer, you must look at the ingredients list. If you notice the term "partially hydrogenated" oil, you know the product has trans fat and you should place it on your "eat very, very seldom" or "never going to touch it" lists

Mono- and polyunsaturated fats have very important health benefits. You can find monounsaturated fats in food products such as olives, avocados, nuts, and olive oil. Polyunsaturated fats can be found in salmon, mackerel, tofu, nuts (specifically walnuts), flax products, and canola oil. There is a link to total body inflammation with the type of fat that you eat, which I discuss in detail in Chapter 6.

Multi-vitamin Use

One of the most common supplements that athletes take is a multi-vitamin. Many athletes use many types of nutrition supplements, such as energy bars, drinks, and gels that contain a good amount of vitamins and minerals. However, what many athletes forget is that these sports nutrition products can sometimes be substituted for pills or powders, depending on the quantity of micronutrients they contain.

FUELTIP

One of my favorite examples involves an athlete with whom I once worked; in addition to having a fairly well-balanced eating program, he consumed more than seven energy bars per day during higher training loads. On top of that, this athlete also took a multivitamin with very high levels of nutrients. I helped this athlete realize that eating seven energy bars per day not only failed to be a helpful nutrition practice, but also that he was overconsuming vitamins and minerals from all of the non-food products that he was taking. The take-home message is that, during certain times of the year (competition season, high-intensity training, two-a-days, etc.), in certain locations (altitude, pollution) or during times of high stress (training load or other life stressors), a good multivitamin containing adequate amounts of nutrients can certainly be helpful in maintaining good health and performance, but athletes must balance their use of other sports nutrition products that also contain high amounts of vitamins and minerals.

The fat-soluble vitamins A, D, E, and K are stored in your body, so taking an enormous amount consistently may lead to developing toxic levels in the future. The water-soluble vitamins B and C are not stored in your body as much, but they should not be taken in excess on a daily, consistent basis because these vitamins do not have much of a storage tank inside the body and are excreted efficiently.

There are some micronutrients, such as iron, sodium, potassium, calcium, copper, iodine, magnesium, manganese, and phosphorus, that are lost through sweat. Because of the high sweat rates of some athletes and the practice of caloric restriction as a way of life for weight-class athletes, it could be reasonable to assume that more micronutrients may be needed at certain times of the training year.

Athletes must be careful not to subscribe to the "more is better" mantra. Overconsuming certain micronutrient supplements or taking individual vitamin and mineral supplements could cause toxicities and possibly deficiencies in other nutrients. Iron is a good example to illustrate this. Many athletes, specifically females, can have low iron stores as a result of poor dietary intake of iron, training status, and the menstrual cycle. I have seen this in many sports from track and field to tennis to triathlon. As you will learn in more detail in Chapter 6, iron is extremely important for the delivery of oxygen to the muscles and is therefore a key nutrient for athletes. However, taking supplemental iron without first having an analysis of blood iron stores may result in an increase in oxidation of cells inside the arteries and can cause deficiencies of other minerals such as zinc and copper.

Variety

Every sport dietitian will tell you to increase the variety of your nutrition plan at some point, and with good reason. More variety means a greater amount of nutrients delivered to the body. Many athletes are creatures of habit, especially those who do not know how to cook. In my experiences, it is usually the younger athletes, but not always, who do not have much culinary experience or who grew up eating convenience foods. These are the athletes who fall victim to leaving out certain foods simply because they either do not know what they are or they do not know how to prepare them. If you overeat in one food group, you do not get all of the essential nutrients that your body needs. For those athletes who are either vegan or vegetarian or who gravitate more toward the carbohydrate-rich foods without a good balance of proteins and healthy fats, blood lipids may be elevated. I have witnessed high triglyceride levels in athletes eating a diet that is too high in carbohydrates for extended periods. This can become a health risk for the athlete. Be sure to mix it up, and choose a variety of foods from all of the food groups. You can easily accomplish this by having lean proteins, color (fruits and vegetables), whole grains, and healthy fats at most meals.

Sharing Nutrition Plans

Each athlete is unique in his or her own way. From genetics to social upbringing, it is important to realize that your body requires different nutrients than your teammate, training partner, or competitor. It is very important not to base your nutrition plan on the needs of somebody else. Nutrition is highly individualized and is based on your health, medical and family history, current fitness level, body-weight goals, and performance-related goals. Your nutrition plan should be as individualized as your training program.

FUELTIP

If I only had a nickel for all of the athletes I have seen fall prey to this one. It's a typical scenario. Athletes want the starting position or see their competitors doing well and want to mimic their routine in order to propel their own performance to that level. They adopt their training program and their eating program. My favorite example of this is an old friend of mine who was a phenomenal triathlete; the night before every sprint triathlon he would compete in, he ate two very large platefuls of fettuccini alfredo. It worked wonders for him because his GI system could handle it and was used to this high-fat meal the night before a race. If I tried that, I would never have made it to the start line. Remember, just because a specific eating program, food, or timing system works for someone else does not mean it works for you. We are all wired differently and require different combinations of nutrients at certain times to maintain a nicely balanced equilibrium within our body.

Most nutrition guidelines for macrocycle eating are fairly well known. However, the difference lies in how the food is used. For athletes with high training loads and frequent competitions, these year-round nutrition concepts become much more important for performance reasons and should be placed as a high priority to lay the nutritional foundation before moving onto the more specific eating strategies of the training cycles presented in the following.

MESOCYCLE AND MICROCYCLE NUTRITION GUIDELINES

Now that you have the overall nutrition goals for the year, let me break down each individual training cycle from a daily, weekly, and monthly perspective. It is very important for you to know when your training volume and/or intensity changes and to correlate that with your nutrition so that you cycle your macro- and micronutrients to support these training load shifts. Remember, the "new school" sports nutrition plans are those that are planned weeks to months in advance rather than during the days leading up to a big competition or training day.

The Pre-season (Preparatory or Base Cycle)

The main nutrition goals of this training cycle include the following:

1. Eat to lose (if appropriate). Pursue active weight loss during this cycle.
1. Eat to train. Eat based on your training load. If your training is beginning lower and building throughout, your nutrition should also follow this same trend.
2. Eat to learn. If you are not trying to lose weight, this is the perfect time to experiment with different foods (not sports nutrition products) throughout the day and during training to determine whether they are "GI friendly" before, during, and after workouts.
3. Eat to improve metabolic efficiency. Teaching the body to use more of its almost unlimited fat stores and to preserve the

very limited carbohydrate stores is a key goal during this training cycle.

This is the training cycle where it all begins again. It is the journey to another competition season. Hopefully, you have taken a bit of time off from structured training and are beginning to build up your volume and intensity slowly. This is extremely beneficial from an injury prevention standpoint, but it also allows you adequate time to adjust your nutrition plan and implement the concept of nutrition periodization. No matter what type of athlete you are, the physiological goals for this training cycle are fairly consistent among most sports: to improve strength, endurance, flexibility, and sometimes sports-specific technical and tactical skills. During this cycle, weight loss may also be a high priority, and rightly so. This is the ideal time to pursue active weight loss. However, this should not be confused with weight cutting for a competition. The active weight loss process has the goal of getting down to a better performance weight before the next training cycle begins. Manipulating your calories for weight loss, that is lowering your calorie intake, will not likely have a negative effect on your performance because you are probably not doing much high-intensity, explosive work in your daily training.

If weight loss is your goal, focus on it in the first three quarters of this training cycle. As you get close to the next training cycle, a lower calorie intake, combined with a bit more volume and intensity being introduced in your training program, may be detrimental to obtaining the higher volume and/or intensity that is required during some training sessions. Remember, the goal of periodizing your training is to provide a smooth progression from one cycle to the next. Active weight loss techniques when intensity begins to increase are not preferred.

The following information provides you with some ranges of nutrients that you can use to help build your eating plan. For qualitative personality types (those who prefer not using many numbers), have no fear. I present a very easy-to-follow qualitative model that is sure to reshape the way you approach food. The best part is that you do not have to count calories or grams!

FUELTIP

This is a great place to mention a topic that is extremely popular among novice athletes. I have had quite a bit experience with those athletes who experience unwanted weight gain during this cycle, specifically in the early portion. I know it may be frustrating because you think that increasing exercise and burning more calories should, at the very least, help maintain your weight, if not create a slight weight loss—but seeing the opposite happen is downright depressing. I am happy to report to you that, nine times out of ten, it is a simple "misunderstanding" of your mind and your body—that is, your ability to realize when you are physically hungry versus psychologically hungry. I discuss these topics in more detail in Chapter 4, but the most common nutrition pitfall when athletes fall prey to this unexpected weight loss is that calorie consumption may be increased. I know it may sound strange, but I have noticed that athletes who experience this mysterious weight gain typically begin using sports nutrition products, such as energy bars, gels, sports drinks, and post-workout beverages, before they need them. Regardless of whether you are trying to lose weight or not, consuming these products in the first part of this training cycle is not needed or recommended unless you are completing glycogen-depleting workouts. These are defined as very high-intensity or very long-duration (over 3 hours) exercise. Certainly there are athletes, such as cyclists, swimmers, rowers, and triathletes, who may train for longer than 3 hours at a time during this cycle and who may actually need the extra calories (from food) during the workout, but, for the others not falling into this category, eating a meal or snack 1–3 hours before the training session and hydrating with water during the session works great.

I should say that I typically get the feedback from athletes indicating that they don't know where they fall in each range. This is a very valid question and one for which I do not have a definite answer. Because eating programs are very specific to each athlete, gender, sport, and position, it is difficult to make individual recommendations in a book format. However, I provide you with tips that you can use to customize your ranges based on your training load and body weight/composition and strength goals. Ultimately, you must customize these to your specific needs and goals.

For the more quantitative personality types (those who prefer numbers), I provide very training cycle-specific quantities of the macronutrients carbohydrate, protein, and fat. As you discovered earlier, the research provides a hefty range of each, but I break these numbers into specific training cycles based on physical goals and energy expenditure. I do my best to represent most sports throughout, but please note that certain sports may have different needs and so more customization is needed.

Daily Nutrition for the Pre-Season: Quantitative Recommendations

Carbohydrate intake should range from 3–7 grams per kilogram of body weight (g/kg) during the pre-season, depending on body weight or composition goals. Additionally, where you fall in this range depends on your sport and position. On the average, use 3–4 g/kg for weight loss goals and 5–7 g/kg for goals without weight loss. $61 \text{ kg} \times 3g = 183g \text{ Carbs} = 732 \text{ cals}.$

FUELTIP

Until volume starts to increase or until you are doing two training sessions per day (strength plus aerobic or aerobic plus aerobic), I recommend that the majority of your carbohydrate consumption comprise fruits and vegetables because they contain beneficial vitamins, minerals, antioxidants, and fiber. A good goal is to eat a minimum of six servings and a maximum of 12 servings of fruits and vegetables per day. I know it sounds somewhat unrealistic, but remember, the serving sizes of fruits and vegetables are fairly small, so if you eat 1–2 servings at every meal and snack, you can easily attain this goal.

FUELTIP

There has been quite a bit of interest in and research about animal protein and health, and there are some fairly good data to suggest that consuming too much animal protein could have a negative effect on health. Much of the data point toward the saturated and trans fat found in some animal proteins. In Chapter 2, I have already discussed the health and performance decrements that these types of fats can have. However, the take-home message is that eating too much moderate to higher-fat animal proteins can negatively affect your health, which could negatively affect your performance. The type of food you eat is your choice, but it is worth mentioning that there have been some very good advances in non-animal protein food sources that can complement your list of animal proteins. Out are the days when tofu was one of the only options—and it definitely did not top most athletes' list of foods. Nowadays there are many great plant-based proteins to choose from that actually taste good and that make it much easier to begin to replace the higher saturated and trans fat animal protein with plant proteins that contain less harmful fat and a better proportion of the healthier fats. I provided some information on these plant-based protein sources in Chapter 2 and go into more detail about them when I discuss vegetarian eating for athletes in Chapter 6. Needless to say, choosing beans, nuts, and soy products is a great option for even the heartiest animal protein eaters because of their wide array of health- and performance-enhancing benefits. Just keep in mind that the fiber content is much higher in plant-based protein sources versus animal-based protein sources; you want to introduce the higher amount of fiber in your eating program gradually to prevent a sudden "shock" to your body.

Protein intake should range from 1.2–2.5 g/kg. It may not seem like this should be such a large range, but, again, your protein intake depends largely on your body weight and composition goals along with your strength training emphasis. If you are in a hypertrophy strength training phase, a range of 1.7–2.0 g/kg can help maintain muscle protein stores. If you are not lifting and do not have much intensity in your workouts, choose a range of 1.2–1.6 g/kg. If you are trying to lose weight or body fat, a shift in macronutrients that includes a slight increase in protein could be justified. You will learn more about the effects of protein for weight loss in Chapter 4, but for this specific goal, a protein range of 2.0–2.5 g/kg could be justified.

Fat intake should range from 0.8–1.3 g/kg. Do not take the lower end of the range to mean that you should go even lower. I know some athletes are fat "phobic," but, as you learned in Chapter 2, your body needs certain types of fat to run smoothly. I recommend, for athletes with weight or body composition goals, a daily fat intake range from 0.8–1.0 g/kg, and, for those in a weight maintenance phase, I recommend consuming 0.9–1.3 g/kg.

FUELTIP

With the obvious health concerns surrounding fat intake, it is best to focus on the healthier mono- and polyunsaturated fats. The benefits are vast, as I described in the previous chapter. Food sources include olives, avocados, fish, nuts, and extra virgin olive oil. Try to decrease the amount of unhealthy saturated fats such as high-fat animal products and less healthy oils. The nutrition facts label on a food product does not always tell the entire story regarding what is actually in the product. This is why it is crucial for you to move your eyes down to the ingredients portion of the food label. Move past the grams and milligrams of nutrients and go straight to what is in the food product, which is where you will learn if any questionable ingredients are in the product.

Fluid

There are no definitive daily hydration guidelines that are supported by research; however, I like to teach athletes how to use a few simple assessment tools to monitor daily hydration status. The first is urine color. The normal color of your urine throughout the day should ideally be pale yellow. Obviously, many factors disrupt this color, such as the first void of the morning and taking supplements, specifically B vitamins. A good rule of thumb is to begin assessing the color of your urine after the first void in the morning.

The second tool is frequency. Urinating every 2–3 hours throughout the day provides a rough indication of hydration status. Urinating too often or not often enough can indicate improper daily hydration techniques. For those who do not like drinking plain water to meet their hydration needs, fruits, vegetables, and other liquids such as milk and tea can be used to hydrate the body.

FUELTIP

Hydration guidelines that include a specific number of cups per day is outdated, as is assuming a portion of your body weight to configure the amount of water you drink. Hydration is very individual; some athletes may require more or less fluid for hydration based on many factors, such as food intake, exercise frequency, intensity, time and type, sweat rate, and geographical location/environmental conditions. One of the most accurate methods of assessing your daily hydration status is by using a refractometer. It is not as technical to do as the term makes it sound. By taking a urine sample first thing in the morning and placing a few drops into the refractometer, you can know your exact urine specific gravity (often referred to as USG), which is a much more accurate method of determining whether you are or are not hydrated. Refractometers are fairly inexpensive, ranging from $80–300, and are easy to use. They are also very easy to travel with because they are normally the size of a cell phone or smaller.

Table 3.1
Summary of Daily Nutrition Needs During the Pre-Season

Training Cycle	CHO	PRO	FAT
Preparatory (no weight loss)	4–7 g/kg	1.2–2.0 g/kg	0.9–1.3 g/kg
Preparatory (for weight loss)	3–4 g/kg	2.0–2.5 g/kg	0.8–1.0 g/kg
	183g	122g	48.8g
	732 cals	488 cals	439 cals

Total = 1659

DAILY NUTRITION FOR THE PRE-SEASON: QUALITATIVE RECOMMENDATIONS

If you really don't want anything to do with the quantitative aspect of nutrition periodization, I understand. In fact, whenever I begin working with an athlete, I never introduce quantitative tools for fear of attrition. I introduce two very simple qualitative methods to athletes that guarantee success because the foundation of using them is understanding food from a satiety standpoint. I prefer to teach athletes how to combine certain foods at certain times to get the most "bang for their buck" without having to count calories or grams. I highly recommend beginning with this step, and, if you decide to progress to the quantitative method, so be it. Using the qualitative tools in the beginning ensures that you have a good foundational knowledge of food before moving to the numbers.

The two qualitative methods that I have developed are the FuelTarget™ and the Periodization Plates™. These are both new additions to this updated edition, and they will not disappoint you. Both work in concert with one another but can also be used independently. I have used both of these tools with many groups of athletes, ranging from kids to Olympic medalists. Their simplicity may confuse you at first because you likely think that nutrition cannot be that easy. It can be, and it is. My mantra, "simple is sustainable," along with the accompanying tools, have awed athletes and coaches alike and continues to prove that once you learn more about your body's response to certain food and its hunger and satiety levels, it is extremely easy to manage it without playing the numbers game.

THE FUELTARGET™

I developed this model to teach athletes how to put foods together to have the most benefit in regards to controlling blood sugar. Much of the work I do with this model is based on listening to the body's hunger signals surrounding meal and snack times.

As can be seen from Figure 3.2, the FuelTarget™ looks like a target or dartboard. There are three areas or rungs that comprise the model; each is associated with a nutrient group. The first rung, or the bulls-eye, is lean protein and healthy fats. The second is fruits and vegetables, and the third is whole grains and healthier starches (nonrefined). This is the foundation of using this model. However, there are little circles on the outside of the FuelTarget™ itself. These "misses," as I call them, are actually key components to using the model and being successful. The misses represent any food or beverage that cannot be placed in the three previously mentioned categories (rungs 1–3). Examples include alcohol, chocolate, candy, pastries, and ice cream. These should be part of a normal nutrition plan, but in minimal amounts. I do not support "cheat" days because they do not teach athletes how to have a good relationship with food. Rather, I promote having controlled misses a few times per week to begin with, in an effort to allow the body to learn to respond to the behavioral aspect of eating these types of foods and beverages.

I know it may sound awkward at first, but remember that changing an eating style is a behavior change, and most research (and my real-life work with athletes) proves that an all-or-nothing approach does not lead to long-term success. Thus, you also see a 90% and 10%, inside and outside the FuelTarget™, respectively. The 90% represents the time to spend inside your personal FuelTarget™ and the 10% represents the amount of misses to allow.

The last explanation of the FuelTarget™ is to "eat from the inside out." Some athletes are guilty of eating from the outside in, which means that they overload their bodies with starchy carbohydrates and consume few fruits, vegetables, lean protein, and healthy fats. In order to be successful in controlling blood sugar, protein and fiber are required in one feeding. Thus, by eating from the inside out, or focusing on putting a lean protein/healthy fat on your plate, followed by a fruit or vegetable and finally a whole grain, you ensure that your blood sugar and insulin levels remain stable throughout the day and provide you with enough energy

FuelTarget™

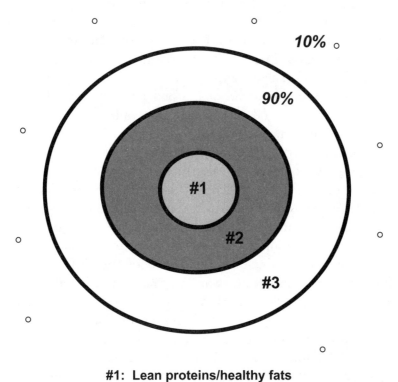

#1: Lean proteins/healthy fats

#2: Fruits and vegetables

#3: Whole grains/healthier starches

○ **"Misses" (keep to 10% or less of the time)**

Figure 3.2

to support training. This is not a recommendation to follow a high-protein eating plan. Rather, my goal is for you to always ask the following questions (in order) when choosing a food: (1) Where is my protein and healthy fat? (2) Where is my color? and (3) Where is my whole grain? By combining foods, you elicit a much more stable blood sugar and insulin response, which has a benefit in enhancing health and improving performance.

You may now be wondering how to use the FuelTarget™. There are no calories or serving sizes, so how on earth can you use something so simple? As mentioned previously, that was my goal when developing this model—to provide a fail-proof, easy-to-use method of delivering nutrition to athletes of all ages. I first developed the model for use with advanced athletes but quickly found that the simplicity suited everyone, even the most analytical athlete type. The beauty about using the FuelTarget™ is that you just have to identify the foods you enjoy to eat in each rung of the model. Refer to the FuelTarget™ Foodlists in Table 3.2 that provide a starter list of foods that belong in each category. You can choose the foods you enjoy from this list and continue to develop your list as your taste preferences change or as you discover new foods. Once you identify your enjoyable foods, it is simply a matter of putting them together based on your palate. Remember, though, eating from the inside out is your first order of business, so when putting together a meal or snack, always choose foods in the order of the FuelTarget™.

There is one additional step in using the FuelTarget™—applying the FuelTarget Zones™ to your specific situation. I developed the FuelTarget Zones™ to combine the simplicity of balancing blood sugar and insulin with my nutrition periodization concept. As you can see from Figure 3.3, the FuelTarget Zones™ highlights specific nutrients to include in your daily nutrition plan based on your training cycle physical demands, weight, and metabolic efficiency goals. The nutrients included on the inside of each zone provide the specific nutrient recommendation based on the zone. For example, Zone 1 includes choosing mostly lean protein, healthy fat, and fruits and vegetables, with the occasional whole

Table 3.2

Lean Protein Sources

Chicken	Beef
Fish	Pork
Turkey	Milk, eggs
Cottage cheese	Cheese (lower fat)
Yogurt	Tofu
Beans	Tempeh
Nuts	Soy milk
Quinoa	Edamame

Fruit and Vegetable Sources

Strawberries	Blueberries
Cantaloupe	Pineapple
Cherries	Blackberries
Kiwi	Oranges
Plums	Peaches
Star fruit	Apples
Pears	Bananas
Broccoli	Kale
Spinach	Asparagus
Sweet potatoes	Cabbage
Bell peppers	Zucchini

Whole Grain Sources

Cereal	Crackers
Tortillas	Bread
Couscous	Quinoa
Oatmeal	Pancakes
Waffles	Bagels
English muffins	Pasta
Rice	Grits

FuelTarget™ and FuelTarget Zones™

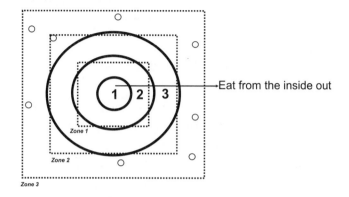

1: lean protein/healthy fat
2: fruits/vegetables
3: whole grains
○: "misses"

Zone 1: Off-season, Weight loss, Metabolic efficiency
Zone 2: Preseason, Competition
Zone 3: Competition or Weight gain

Figure 3.3

grain. Zone 2 includes lean protein, healthy fat, fruits and vegetables, and whole grains, with more allowable misses, whereas Zone 3 includes all of the previously mentioned nutrients.

I encourage athletes to follow Zone 1 when they are in an off-season, if they seek weight loss, and for improving metabolic efficiency. Zone 2 is used during the pre-season and for some athletes during competition, while Zone 3 is typically used for athletes who need to gain weight.

You may have noticed that I have not specified the quantity to eat while using the FuelTarget™. Because this is a qualitative model, I do not like to focus on using numbers in the implementation strategy. By simply grouping the nutrients together in the "eat from the inside out" rule, your satiety is improved throughout the day. A clear-cut way of knowing if you are putting the proper quantities of the nutrients together in one feeding is to assess your biological hunger response. I discuss this in more detail in Chapter

4, but in brief, the nutrients you eat should keep you full for approximately 3–4 hours. If they do not, simply increase the portions from left to right from the FuelTarget™ Foodlist.

THE PERIODIZATION PLATES™

I have developed another model that complements the FuelTarget™ and can be used together or interchangeably depending on your personal preferences. This model, called the Periodization Plates™, is another simple, qualitative tool that you can use to learn the proper foods to eat based on your training cycle. As you can see from figure 3.4, the Periodization Plates™ model uses a normal plate as an example of how to proportion the different nutrients (what I call macronutrient shifting) on the plate based on your training cycle. It is made up of four nutrient categories: (1) lean protein/healthy fat, (2) fruits and vegetables, (3) whole grains, and (4) sports nutrition products

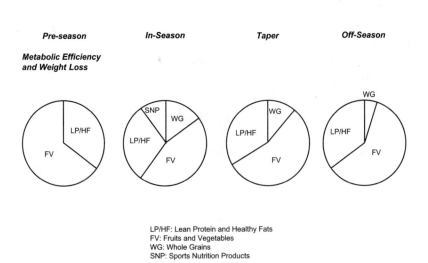

Figure 3.4

(which are considered misses when using the FuelTarget™). Each nutrient category is shifted to include more or less, based on your training cycle and training load changes throughout the year.

It is important to realize that the Periodization Plates™ simply acts as a guide for you to use. The four different examples represent the general shifts in nutrients; there is not one Periodization Plates™ model that is the only option that you should use. They are provided as a reference point to provide you a visual representation of how to portion the food that you eat.

The Periodization Plates™ can be customized based on body weight goals and energy expenditure. A goal of weight loss includes a higher amount of lean protein/healthy fat to improve satiety; a moderate amount of fruits and vegetables to supply necessary carbohydrates, vitamins, minerals, and phytochemicals; and a lower amount of whole grains. For weight gain, lean protein/healthy fat portion is the same as for weight loss, but portions of fruits and vegetables are reduced, with servings of whole grains increased to account for higher calorie needs. This is just one example of how to use nutrition periodization to customize your nutrition plan based on body weight goals.

Another very important point as it relates to using the Periodization Plates™ is to utilize different plates on different days to account for training load changes. For example, if you have an intense or longer-duration workout, the in-season plate can be used. If you have a recovery day or lighter training day, it could be possible to use the pre-season plate. I term this "microcycle periodization," and the purpose of using it is to customize your nutrition plan fully in an effort to use nutrition to support physical energy demands.

Similar to the FuelTarget™, the Periodization Plates™ is a qualitative model and should not include numbers. Implementing a daily nutrition plan properly using the Periodization Plates™ is as simple as trying to mimic closely the plate pattern listed under each training cycle. You body self-regulates once you reteach it to listen to its hunger and satiety cues again. There is almost always a break-in period, which I normally consider to be 3–7 days.

During this time, explore how much of a food is needed to affect your hunger response and for you to remain full.

As mentioned previously, the main goal of combining foods in this manner by using the Periodization Plates™ is to maintain blood sugar for at least 3 hours. If you eat a meal and get hungry in less than that amount of time, or if you want to lose weight or body fat, I recommend that you increase your lean protein/healthy fat portion by 50–75% at each meal in order to have a more profound affect on satiety. You will likely undereat and overeat during this time. Expect it. It happens, but it is a positive step in terms of being more in tune with your body and listening to the cues related to hunger. In a short time, you will know how to combine foods properly to have the best satiety effect, and you will know when your body requires nourishment.

TRAINING NUTRITION FOR THE PRE-SEASON

Specific nutrient timing protocols should be used before, during, and after training sessions. However, it is important to keep in mind that these also change and are periodized based on your specific training cycle. Your body requires more or less nutrients surrounding a training session, depending on the type, duration, and intensity of workouts and your overall physical goals for this cycle.

Before Training

Fluid

Hydration tops the list for sustaining and improving performance in athletes. One of the most important and often forgotten goals is to hydrate well throughout the day to prepare for your training session(s). Current recommendations include drinking 0.07–0.10 ounces of fluid (preferably water in most cases) 4 hours before training and an additional 0.04–0.10 ounces 2 hours before training if you are not fully hydrated.

> **FUELTIP**
>
> Since the first edition of this book was published, fluid guidelines have been updated by the American College of Sports Medicine. The new position paper on Exercise and Fluid Replacement (2007) bases fluid intake on body weight rather than providing an absolute range. Although this may seem a bit more confusing and tedious to determine proper hydration guidelines, it is much better for athletes, because it is based on body weight and we know that body weight can fluctuate significantly among athletes from workout to workout. I have constructed an easy chart, Table 3.3, for these new fluid strategies so you don't have to break out the calculator. Refer to it to customize your fluid needs fully before a training session or race.

Don't let the numbers confuse you. The main reason for the emphasis on pre-training fluid intake is to prevent dehydration throughout the workout. If you can pre-hydrate your body well enough, you minimize the amount of fluids that you lose during a training session; therefore, you can recover your fluid stores more efficiently and not be forced to drink much afterward. It may not seem like it until you actually try it, but it is a win-win situation.

For athletes with early morning practices, it is extremely difficult to be fully hydrated before the training session. In these cases, I recommend that the athlete begin the rehydration process by drinking small amounts of fluids that contain electrolytes (specifically sodium) that are tolerated well by the gut and can be held down during the workout. Water, although it is a good beverage, is not the best rehydrating choice; thus athletes should not over-consume water without eating food or consuming electrolytes. Juice, lemonade, milk, or a smoothie can be used in small quantities in the early morning to begin the rehydration process.

Carbohydrates

It is obviously important to consume carbohydrates before a training session, but if this training cycle does not have high-energy

Table 3.3
Hydration Table, Based on Body Weight

Body Weight	Ounces of fluid based on 0.04	Ounces of fluid based on 0.07	Ounces of fluid based on 0.10
100	4.0	7	10.0
105	4.2	7.4	10.5
110	4.4	7.7	11.0
115	4.6	8.1	11.5
120	4.8	8.4	12.0
125	5.0	8.8	12.5
130	5.2	9.1	13.0
135	5.4	9.5	13.5
140	5.6	9.8	14.0
145	5.8	10.2	14.5
150	6.0	10.5	15.0
155	6.2	10.9	15.5
160	6.4	11.2	16.0
165	6.6	11.6	16.5
170	6.8	11.9	17.0
175	7.0	12.3	17.5
180	7.2	12.6	18.0
185	7.4	13.0	18.5
190	7.6	13.3	19.0
195	7.8	13.7	19.5
200	8.0	14.0	20.0
205	8.2	14.4	20.5
210	8.4	14.7	21.0
215	8.6	15.1	21.5
220	8.8	15.4	22.0
225	9.0	15.8	22.5
230	9.2	16.1	23.0
235	9.4	16.5	23.5
240	9.6	16.8	24.0
245	9.8	17.2	24.5
250	10.0	17.5	25.0
255	10.2	17.9	25.5
260	10.4	18.2	26.0
265	10.6	18.6	26.5
270	10.8	18.9	27.0
275	11.0	19.3	27.5
280	11.2	19.6	28.0
285	11.4	20.0	28.5
290	11.6	20.3	29.0
295	11.8	20.7	29.5
300	12.0	21.0	30.0

expenditure demands in terms of long-duration or high-intensity workouts, a snack or small feeding will more than provide your body with the nutrients it needs. The form of carbohydrate largely depends on your sport and training session. For example, runners may fair better at consuming a small smoothie or glass of juice because of the digestive problems experienced sometimes with the up and down movement of running. Contact sports, such as boxing, wrestling, football, and martial arts would also fall into this category because of the possibility of the athlete being hit or thrown. In contrast, athletes such as cyclists, baseball players, golfers, and sailors may be able to introduce a more solid source of carbohydrate to their pre-workout plan because of the more stable digestive process of their sport. Of course, all athletes should be treated individually and should customize their pre-workout carbohydrate consumption based on the daily training goals. Liquid sources of carbohydrates are much easier and quicker to digest, followed by semi-solid sources and lastly, solid sources.

FUELTIP

Because you wake up in a dehydrated state, I normally recommend scheduling non-quality training sessions in the early morning if at all possible. Workouts that are technique- or aerobic-focused should be the goal because you likely wake up in a negative performance hydration state.

It is normally recommended to consume roughly 1–4 grams of carbohydrate per kilogram of body weight 1–4 hours before a training session. For a 180–pound athlete, this equals roughly 82–327 grams or 328–1308 calories. However, I have found that although this is what current sports nutrition research recommends, if you teach your body to become more metabolically efficient, you can lower your pre-workout carbohydrate needs. Regardless of quantity, it is still important to provide your body with carbohydrate sources before training. Just the quantity differs based on the training session, your body weight/ composition goals, and how efficient you are at using fat as fuel.

Metabolic efficiency is the relationship of carbohydrate oxidation to fat oxidation throughout different intensities of exercise. As the intensity of exercise increases, the body relies more on carbohydrate as energy. The goal for most athletes should be to improve metabolic efficiency by utilizing fat as energy through a wide range of intensities. This can be done by introducing aerobic training and by consuming a balanced daily nutrition plan that does not provide an overabundance of carbohydrates when the body does not need them.

Aerobic training induces cellular changes that improve the body's efficiency in using macronutrients, specifically fats. Mitochondria increase in size and number as a result of aerobic training. Mitochondrial enzymatic activity also increases—more specifically, those associated with the Kreb's Cycle and respiratory chain, the shuttle system that transfers protons developed through glycolysis into the mitochondria for use in the respiratory chain and fatty acid metabolism. This is important because it allows the body to use more available fats for energy to fuel exercise. The oxidation of fat by the mitochondria is the main source of energy when exercise intensity is low.

Metabolic efficiency can be further manipulated through proper nutrition periodization and timing. It has been known for sometime that eating a higher carbohydrate diet leads to an increase in carbohydrate oxidation. This decreases the body's ability to oxidize fat at higher intensities because of the higher insulin response and accompanying inhibition of lipolysis (the breakdown of fat). Therefore, to properly teach the body to use fat more efficiently, carbohydrate intake should be lower in the beginning of this training cycle. This is not a recommendation to follow a low-carbohydrate diet. Rather, the goal is to balance carbohydrate, protein, and fat intake so that proper metabolic changes can happen.

Early morning workouts are definitely worth mentioning because they are so common and cause nutritional challenges for athletes. Upon waking, you can lose up to 3% of your body weight as fluid, as well as having up to 40% less glycogen (carbohydrate) stores. This puts your body in a dehydrated and somewhat malnourished state when you first roll out of bed. If you have an early morning training session, it is critical that you consume some sort of fluids and electrolytes at a minimum, and a small amount of carbohydrates, if possible, beforehand. A little goes a long ways. After the workout, you can eat a good, well-balanced feeding and fill up your tanks more efficiently.

FUELTIP

There is absolutely no good reason to follow a carbohydrate-loading regimen prior to any workout during this training cycle, especially in the beginning of the cycle, regardless of your body weight or composition goals. If your training load is not high, you do not need this large amount of carbohydrates. Loading your body with excess carbohydrate causes your body to burn more carbohydrate, which means that you will not be able to tap into your fat reserves as efficiently.

Protein

The next nutrient of concern in the pre-training window is protein. The long and the short of it is that not much protein is needed—just enough to help stabilize blood sugar levels. Of course, it depends on the sport and training session goal, whether aerobic- or anaerobic-based, but I normally recommend a range of 5–20 grams of protein in this pre-workout timeframe. I stray on the high end before strength training sessions, to improve protein stores going into the workout, and on the low end for more aerobic- or interval-based training (if this is performed during this cycle). Protein takes a bit longer to digest, so be careful not to consume too much.

Fat

The guidelines for fat are somewhat similar to those for protein. For athletes with sensitive stomachs or those who have contact practices or shorter-endurance training, fat intake prior to training should be minimized. Fat has a slower digestion rate; thus, if you are going to include fat in your pre-training feeding, I recommend lower quantities.

Sodium

Including sodium in the 1–4 hours before a training session is crucial to many athletes for the most important role of aiding in fluid balance. A small amount of sodium is needed in the pre-training feeding. I normally recommend about 500 milligrams with some type of fluid and/or food.

FUELTIP

Acute sodium loading has been proven to reduce urinary output, increase plasma volume, and reduce thermoregulatory strain. Many athletes who have high sweat rates and are competing in warm environments or longer-endurance events have had great success with this type of loading. The protocol can be initiated the night before a training session by consuming 3,500–4,500 milligrams of sodium in frequent doses (every 15–20 minutes) with water (just enough to "wash" down the sodium taste). I recommend this be done in a 3- to 4-hour period after dinner and before bedtime. This can also be replicated in the 2–3 hours before training; however, I normally recommend following this acute sodium loading protocol the night before and then consuming between 800–1,500 milligrams of sodium in the 2- to 3-hour period before training to reduce any possible GI distress.

During Training

It is important to reiterate that this training cycle does not normally have a very high training load in terms of volume or intensity. The most important nutrition goal is hydration. Although it is important to provide the body with the calories necessary for energy, overconsuming carbohydrates works against the metabolic efficiency goals of the athlete. Thus, carbohydrate supplementation should only be used in the following situations:

1. Early morning practice sessions that last longer than 2 hours
2. Training sessions later in the day that last longer than 3 hours.

The most important consideration to facilitate improved metabolic efficiency is to have the well-balanced nutrient feeding before training so that the body is in a well-fed and hydrated state. Especially during this training cycle, this minimizes the need for supplemental carbohydrate during a workout. Because the body has enough stored carbohydrate to fuel about 2–3 hours of moderately intense exercise, it is not necessary to overfeed the body during exercise in the pre-season.

Fluid

There is good research to support drinking 3–8 ounces of fluid every 15–20 minutes during training. This research is what is known as "drinking ahead of thirst." However, emerging theories and questions challenge this research, suggesting that drinking according to thirst—not ahead of thirst—is more beneficial. These theories, based on the work of Dr. Tim Noakes, a physician and exercise physiologist in South Africa, are based on normal physiological responses in the body. In fact, he has noted in research that consuming less fluid per hour results in similar performance markers, such as a lack of differences in core temperature or finishing times. Interestingly, he has found that drinking the higher amount of fluid resulted in some athletes having GI distress. Dr. Noakes's recommendations for hourly fluid intake range from 13.5–27 ounces. If this is split into 15-minute segments, it equates with drinking just over 3 ounces to just under 7 ounces, aligning closely with the recommendations that have been noted in past sports nutrition research. However, the main difference lies in drinking ad libitum, or when you are thirsty. There may be some instances where you may not have to hydrate (in training less than 1 hour), or, based on the workout itself, you may consume less than this amount per hour. It is important that you constantly assess your body instead of trying to drink ahead of schedule. This can result in hyperhydration and the dilution of the body's electrolytes.

The main take-home message with respect to drinking fluids during training is that you should develop good instinct and listen to your body's senses and react to them and adjust accordingly. Learning your body now leads to better hydration management strategies when environmental conditions become warmer and the intensity of training increases, thus causing your body to produce more heat.

Carbohydrate

Scientific research states that athletes should consume between 30–90 grams of carbohydrate per hour of exercise. However, research does not account for the periodization of sport and the ever-varying training load changes that athletes undergo. The concept of nutrition periodization takes this into account and appropriately bases corresponding training nutrition on the physical goals of your individual training sessions.

Thus during this training cycle, where volume and intensity are not too high yet, it is extremely important not to overfeed the body during training sessions that do not require a continuous feeding of sugar. In fact, because the body stores enough carbohydrate to fuel at least 2–3 hours of moderate intense exercise, if your training consists of low-to-moderate volume and intensity and you followed the pre-training nutrition recommendations provided earlier, there may be little reason to consume supplemental carbohydrates during these shorter workouts. Of course, there are exceptions. If you train first thing in the morning without eating anything, it is beneficial to have a little carbohydrate during training lasting longer than 1 hour. Additionally, if your training session lasts longer than about 2 1/2–3 hours, supplemental carbohydrate is needed.

Protein

The latest research has looked at the importance of including protein during training to decreasing muscle soreness and damage following training. Although there is not an exact protein protocol to follow during training, I normally recommend a range of 3–10 grams per hour, depending on your sport and the duration of your training session. If the duration is under 2 hours of training, you likely will not require any protein as long as you eat a good balance of nutrients beforehand.

Fat

It is very unlikely that an athlete will require eating any fat during a workout during this training cycle. However, I have known athletes who are training for longer than 3 hours (usually ultra-endurance runners and cyclists) to consume trail mix with nuts, which are a form of fat. Again, duration somewhat dictates this, but there are no set recommendations of how much fat to consume during a training session. Most athletes do not need to worry about eating fat during a workout at this time of the year.

Sodium

The quantity of sodium needed during training is, by far, one of the most controversial topics and will continue to be. Because this is the pre-season, specific guidelines are not introduced yet. Rather, a small amount of sodium that promotes fluid balance is the goal for athletes to consume during training that lasts longer than 1 hour or is done in a warmer environment. I normally recommend 300–500 milligrams per hour to sustain fluid balance. The next training cycle yields more specific research and application ranges because it pertains to consuming sodium during training.

After Training

I am often asked by athletes during this training cycle why they may be experiencing weight gain (I am not referring to lean muscle mass). Because of media influence and good marketing strategies, athletes often use post-workout powders and bars in the first 30–60 minutes following training sessions. However, this is not necessary for all athletes. Although there are exceptions, because most athletes do not engage in glycogen-depleting exercise (defined as high intensity or longer than 3 hours in duration), using sports nutrition supplements after training is neither necessary nor recommended. The main reason many athletes gain weight (body fat mostly) during this training cycle is because they overconsume calories following mostly aerobic or mildly intense workouts. The truth of the matter is that if you enter a training session well-fueled with a balance of nutrients, you do not need the high calorie option of sports products. Rather, I recommend consuming a light snack or meal if it can be coordinated around a meal time. If eating a snack, a repeat of your pre-workout snack will suffice. For example, if you had a glass of a milk-based fruit smoothie before training, have another glass of it following training. It is that easy and does not introduce too many calories when your body simply does not need them.

Fluid

Good research supports the fact that, for proper rehydration, 150% of fluid losses should be consumed in the 30- to 60-minute "window of opportunity" following training sessions. This is applicable during this training cycle, and athletes should drink 24 ounces of fluid for every pound of body weight that is lost during training. For athletes with a high sweat rate, who lose more than 3 pounds per hour, fluid intake pre-training and during training is of utmost importance. For most athletes, it is difficult to drink more than 24 ounces of fluid after a workout. In fact, too much fluid without adequate sodium could result in hampered rehydration.

Carbohydrate

As mentioned previously, a large amount of carbohydrate is not needed after training if it was not too long or of high intensity. A small snack that consists of at least 20–30 grams of carbohydrate will suffice. It is even better if athletes can time their training session to end before a meal. Remember, overfeeding the body with unnecessary calories leads to unwanted weight and/or body fat gain.

Protein

Similar to carbohydrate, not much protein is needed after most workouts during this training cycle with the exception of strength training sessions. For these, at least 20 grams of protein should be consumed afterward to ensure proper protein balance. For all other training, including technique, aerobic, and nonglycogen-depleting, I recommend a snack of between 5–10 grams of protein to hold the athlete off until mealtime.

Fat

Fat interferes somewhat with carbohydrate absorption; thus a large amount of fat consumed in the first 30–60 minutes following training is not highly recommended. However, a small amount of fat can be consumed when combined with protein and carbohydrate—for example, yogurt, milk, lean meat, or nuts. Minimize the saturated and trans fat intake as much as possible during this time.

Sodium

The amount of sodium to consume after training is important to promote rehydration. I normally recommend about 500 milligrams for athletes to consume through foods such as crackers, pretzels, yogurt, and bread.

In-Season (Competition)

For most athletes, I recommend the following nutrition goals that correspond to the higher-energy expenditure needs:

1. Warming up the gut. Each sport and position requires different body positions, and warming up the gut simply means identifying the food and drink that sit best in the digestive tract before training. Because the intensity of training is increasing, blood flow is minimized in the digestive tract

(shunted to the working muscles), which means less efficient digestion. The food that you ate before your training sessions in the previous cycle may not work the same now that you are training more intensely.

2. Practicing competition simulation eating during training. The stress hormone response encountered at the beginning of a competition sometimes alters certain body responses, such as digestion. It is extremely important to account for this as much as possible by placing a few training sessions at competition intensity, where the specific nutrition plan (before, during, and after) can be tried.

3. Continuing the "less is more" implementation strategy of metabolic efficiency. Although it is true that your body likely requires more carbohydrate during training sessions, if you teach your body how to oxidize more fat during workouts during the pre-season, you will not want to revert to past behaviors and consume a very high carbohydrate diet during training or competition. Because you are more metabolically efficient, you can navigate this higher-intensity training with fewer calories per hour.

4. Fine-tuning your nutrition plan, specifically hydration and electrolytes, based on the environment and length of training session. If you compete in different, challenging environments and durations, your hydration and electrolyte plan may have to change. Although it may be slight, it should be factored in during your more intense training sessions to test the waters before competition rolls around.

5. Avoiding temptations. These, very simply, are mostly related to travel. Because your routine and schedule are disrupted, it is easy to stray from your normal nutrition plan. It is very important to avoid this; take the time to plan and prepare your nutrition plan before traveling. Be sure to locate grocery stores and restaurants and bring any cooking and power devices and food you may need in order to be self-sufficient.

This training cycle progresses into offering more sports-specific goals, such as improving strength, speed, power, force, agility, and economy. Training sessions are much more focused on specificity, and intensity is higher; thus energy expenditure is greater. Because of this, the nutrients that your body needs are different, and the mantra "eat to train, don't train to eat" becomes very important. Going into training sessions well-fueled and hydrated is crucial because it will have a profound effect on how quickly your body can recover from the more challenging workouts.

FUELTIP

Because training sessions are of higher quality during this cycle, it is important to match nutrient intake with the daily training patterns of your program. This microcycle periodization should account for higher and lower training load days, and your nutrition plan should support this. For example, if you have a high-quality, longer than 3 hours training day (as one session or split into different sessions) one day, but a recovery day the next day when you are doing mostly aerobic or technique for less than 1 hour—your daily carbohydrate intake needs to change to support your energy expenditure fluctuations. Additionally, some athletes put in consecutive days of quality training before recovery sessions are planned. Regardless of the pattern, it is important to treat each training day individually and to eat for that day's energy expenditure goals.

Quantitative Recommendations

Daily carbohydrate intake should range from 5–12 g/kg during this cycle. The range is large because it accounts for the quantity of training. For athletes training fewer than 3 hours per day, a range of 5–8 g/kg can be used; athletes training more than 3 hours per day may require a higher intake of 9–12 g/kg.

Protein intake should range from 1.4 to 2.0 g/kg. The lower end can be followed during times of competition, when there is not much training for improved physiological adaptation

Table 3.3
Summary of Daily Nutrition Needs during the Competition Mesocycle

Training Cycle	CHO	PRO	FAT
Competition	5–12 g/kg	1.4–2.0 g/kg	1.0–1.5 g/kg

planned, and the higher end can be followed when you have a good training block leading up to or between competitions.

Fat intake should range from 1.0 to 1.5 g/kg. Most athletes find themselves only needing the lower end of this range, but, for endurance and ultra-endurance athletes and for weight-gain athletes, a higher amount of daily fat may be necessary to maintain energy stores and support body weight goals.

Fluid

Similar to the pre-season, in-season athletes should monitor their daily hydration by the color and frequency of urination. Because of the higher intensity and duration of training sessions, the body may lose more fluids, so it is very important to note that your daily hydration strategy will likely increase from that in the pre-season. Additionally, athletes in some sports may be training more outdoors in more stressful, environmental conditions that increase sweat rate.

Qualitative Recommendations: The FuelTarget™

Training intensity has increased and energy expenditure is greater on some days during this cycle. Using the principles of the FuelTarget™ still applies in terms of eating from the inside out, with the primary goal of stabilizing blood sugar. In fact, it is crucial that you do not abandon all of the great metabolic efficiency work that you did in your prior training cycle. However, because of the greater energy demands, your body may require more nutrients at certain times to supply energy and replenish the stores lost during training. Thus, in terms of the FuelTarget Zones™, it is beneficial now to toggle between Zone 1, when you have a recovery or easier training day or as you are tapering for a competition, and Zone 2, when you have a quality training session or more than two workouts in one day. Following Zone 2 provides your body with extra carbohydrates from whole grains and healthier starches to support these greater energy demands. For athletes who need to keep weight on or gain weight during this training cycle, Zone 3 should be used because it includes a larger volume of foods and helps achieve these body weight goals much more easily.

The following are some examples of daily meals fitting in each of the FuelTarget™ Zones:

FuelTarget™ Zone 1

Breakfast: Scrambled eggs with mushrooms, bell peppers, and tomatoes

Lunch: Spinach salad with carrots, cucumbers, tomato, sunflower seeds, black beans, and chicken pieces

Dinner: Lean steak with broccoli and cauliflower

Snacks: Cottage cheese with fruit

FuelTarget™ Zone 2

Breakfast: Plain yogurt, blueberries, strawberries, granola

Lunch: Turkey sandwich with lettuce, tomato, mustard, with an apple and cottage cheese

Dinner: Salmon with asparagus and quinoa

Snack: Trail mix with mixed nuts, raisins, and carob chips

FuelTarget™ Zone 3

Breakfast: Smoothie with milk, fruit, and whey protein powder; whole grain toast with peanut butter; bowl of whole grain cereal with milk

Lunch: Buffalo burger with sweet potato wedges, mixed vegetables, and a milkshake

Dinner: Chicken fajitas with bell peppers, cheese, black beans, and guacamole; brown rice

Snacks: Pistachios with crackers and cheese

The Periodization Plates™

The Periodization Plates™ can also be used as a model to guide your eating during this training cycle, but the next progression, the in-season plate, should be used. Additionally, for athletes who are tapering (reducing volume and maintaining or slightly increasing intensity) for a competition, the taper plate should be used in the days or weeks leading up to a competition, but only when the formal taper is implemented.

The use of sports nutrition products are beneficial during this time of the training year but should not be abused and should not replace normal meals. They can be used for additional snacks or surrounding a training session.

FUELTIP

Intensity of exercise can significantly change the digestive functioning of your gut. Because of this and the higher stress hormone response, it is important to find a liquid source of electrolytes and calories because this is likely easier for your body to process before a high-intensity workout or competition. Try a series of liquid sources in high-quality training sessions that exude some form of high pressure to complete in order to stimulate the stress response similar to that on competition day.

TRAINING NUTRITION FOR THE COMPETITION SEASON

This training cycle likely includes higher-intensity strength training, longer endurance, and greater power and force workouts. Your training week is likely separated into specific quality versus non-quality sessions to account for proper physical adaptation and recovery. This microcycle periodization can be somewhat challenging from a fueling perspective, because you want to obtain a balance between underfeeding your body and overfeeding it before, during, and after workouts.

Before Training

Fluid

Somewhat similar hydration goals exist before a training session during this cycle as they did in the pre-season. However, there are a few special considerations. First, environmental conditions may be different. If the weather is warmer and more humid, fluid needs likely increase because of increased sweat rates. Second, it is common to have more frequent early morning workouts, and competitions can also be held in the mornings with some sports. This makes pre-hydrating a bit of a challenge; thus, although it may not be realistic to follow the fluid recommendations recommended in the pre-season cycle, it is important to begin the hydration process before the competition. This can be done by drinking 12–20 ounces of a fluid that has carbohydrate and sodium, with possibly a small amount of protein.

FUELTIP

I should mention the concept of eating "clean." Some athletes make a conscious effort to reduce the processed foods and focus on fruits, vegetables, leaner proteins and animal products, and nonrefined whole grains. This is a very healthy method of eating; however, if you follow an eating program similar to this, remember that, because of the increased nutrient density, you will feel fuller longer and you may not be that hungry throughout the day. This can actually produce unnecessary weight loss because of the higher nutrient density and lower calorie intake combined with the increased energy expenditure with higher-intensity training. One of the best methods I have used with athletes who have a hard time maintaining weight during this cycle while eating "clean" is to provide 1–2 milk-based fruit smoothies per day with a good amount of carbohydrate and protein and a splash of healthy fat.

Carbohydrates

It is important to consider the goal of the training session and the time of the workout before planning your nutrition. Because your body is in a relatively fasted and somewhat dehydrated state upon waking, eat and drink something to get the nourishment and hydration process started again, especially if you will be doing a quality workout. Ideally, the quality workout would not fall within 2–3 hours upon waking, but, if it needs to happen sooner, at least try to replenish some of your fluid stores by drinking a bit of fruit juice with a small pinch of salt, or better yet, if your stomach can handle it, a fruit smoothie made with some type of milk (cow's, rice, almond, soy) or a little whey protein isolate powder. However, if you have an aerobic training session planned early in the morning that is less than 2 hours in length, you can likely get by without eating anything until afterward. If you wake up hungry, listen to your body and feed it with a small, macronutrient-balanced snack. But if you simply are not hungry that early in the morning, introduce a fluid source during the workout and eat a balanced breakfast afterward.

If you do not have a morning training session, you can follow similar carbohydrate intake guidelines as presented in the previous training cycle (1–4 grams of carbohydrate per kilogram of body weight, 1–4 hours before a training session).

However, carbohydrate loading is not beneficial for all athletes, especially those competing in weight class sports (wrestlers, boxers, some martial arts). For most athletes who are not competing in longer-duration and higher-intensity events, following a moderate carbohydrate daily eating plan is more than sufficient to have enough carbohydrate stores prior to competition. In addition, some research has suggested that carbohydrate loading is more beneficial for males than females. Because of different hormonal responses, females may benefit more from eating carbohydrates during a competition than from trying to store more beforehand.

If you choose to carbohydrate load, it is important to know that there are many protocols in existence. A 24-hour carbo-hydrate loading protocol has been shown to be just as beneficial as the traditional 5- to 7-day protocol. I think this is fantastic news for many reasons. First and foremost is that with an increase in carbohydrate consumption typically comes an increase in body weight. Most athletes I have worked with see this as a negative contributor to performance, especially because it falls during a taper, or lower-volume week. Even though the body stores more carbohydrate and, consequently, more water, athletes typically feel "heavy" and sometimes lethargic.

FUELTIP

Carbohydrate loading has been proven to be of great benefit, mostly for endurance athletes or athletes who are competing at higher intensities in many events throughout the day (swimmers, baseball players, and some track athletes) or those competing in events longer than 3 hours (tennis and football players).

Second, a 1-day loading protocol has merit in terms of travel schedules. Food at competition venues often is not similar to what the athletes have been eating in their normal routine; thus, trying to eat more carbohydrates from less common foods for 5–7 days may cause GI distress. Loading for 1-day, by eating 10 grams of carbohydrate per kilogram of body weight, can be done by simply packing carbohydrate-rich foods, such as pasta, rice, potatoes, and oatmeal, that can be easily cooked in a hot pot in a hotel room.

However, to play devil's advocate, I will state that the only negative that could be associated with this 1-day loading protocol is slower digestion. As mentioned in Chapter 2, it takes between 24–72 hours for food to go from entry to exit in the body. If you eat too many carbohydrates the day before a competitive event, the food may not be fully digested by the time competition begins.

As a sports dietitian, I have to be sensitive to different athletes and sports. I believe the 24-hour carbohydrate loading protocol has great merit for those athletes who already follow a fairly high-carbohydrate eating plan. This day of loading before competition is not really loading for these athletes. However, for those who follow a significantly lower-carbohydrate eating plan, 1-day loading may not be enough to fill glycogen stores. Even more important, if athletes double or even triple their carbohydrate intake in 1 day, their GI system may not fully agree, and stomach issues such as bloating, gas, or possible constipation may arise.

For weight-class sport athletes, weight cutting is often the norm, and these athletes typically have only a few hours after weigh-in to attempt to rehydrate and refuel. Although this is not considered carbohydrate loading, I recommend that these athletes consume an adequate amount of fluid and food with a higher sodium and carbohydrate content.

Some athletes are concerned with how much carbohydrate is needed in a loading phase if they are already following a high-carbohydrate eating plan. Normally, if you consume fewer than 10 grams of carbohydrate per kilogram of body weight on a daily basis, a carbohydrate loading regimen may be of benefit to you. However, if you consume more than 10 grams per kilogram, simply maintain this amount leading up to your competition.

If you choose to load on carbohydrates either 1 day or 1 week before competition, be psychologically ready for the associated consequences, such as weight gain. More carbohydrate stores in your body lead to more water storage, and, even though this may be good for performance, you must be prepared for it mentally. I have witnessed far too many athletes who are caught off guard during this time and whose psyche is temporarily "damaged" because of this associated weight gain. This is definitely not the proper pre-competition mental zone to be in before an important competition.

Protein

Most of the protein recommendations before training during this higher-intensity cycle are based on the type of workout. Normally, it is not a good idea to consume too much protein before a workout because of the slower digestion rate. However, for strength workouts, where the goal of maintaining the body's protein stores becomes a priority, eating 20–25 grams of protein can assist in preventing significant protein degradation during the workout.

FUELTIP

You may have heard of those athletes with "iron stomachs." In fact you may be one of those lucky athletes! In these situations, I don't think it is too important to implement a fiber taper because you will likely not experience any GI distress. However, if you are an athlete who has a fairly sensitive stomach that becomes even more so when stress hormones are elevated before a competition, it may be a good idea to follow a short fiber taper to allow less residue in your GI tract and less chance of taking bathroom breaks during your competition. If you choose a fiber taper, begin decreasing your total fiber intake 2–3 days before the competition. A good stepwise progression is to decrease total fiber by 50% on the first day and then by 25% on the subsequent days. To accomplish this most efficiently, decrease the amount of fruit, vegetables, and whole grains that you eat. Make special note of sports nutrition supplements during this time also. Many companies produce products, specifically energy bars, that have a more healthy nutrient profile with higher fiber. Good low-fiber foods include fruit and vegetable juices, white bread, and canned goods. I know these suggestions are not high on the healthy meter, but you only eat them for a very short time. It won't be long enough to develop into a habit or have adverse health consequences. However, it is extremely important for you to try this in training first because a rapid switch to a low-fiber diet could result in constipation or hemorrhoids. I have said it before and will again, customize this to your body. A lower-fiber diet may or may not be right for you. You know your body better than anyone.

Aside from that type of workout, a high amount of protein before training is not necessary. A range of 5–15 grams will suffice and should be based on what your digestive system can handle beforehand.

Fat

The guidelines for fat are somewhat similar to those of protein. A little fat can be consumed before training, but it should be based on the individual gut response. Additionally, if fat is to be eaten, the right type is of extreme importance. As mentioned in the previous chapter, certain fats can increase inflammation in the body. This is not a good thing, especially before a training session. Thus, limiting saturated and trans fats in the 1- to 2-hour window before training is beneficial. Mono- and polyunsaturated fats are the preferred sources.

Sodium

Using sodium in the pre-workout time is even more important during this training cycle to help maintain fluid stores, but it also helps in nerve impulse transmission and muscular contraction. Be sure to include a good source of sodium through food or beverage in the 30–90 minutes leading up to a training session. And remember, acute sodium loading, as presented in the pre-season information, can be extremely useful during this training cycle.

During Training

It is very easy to reverse the metabolic efficiency state that you created in your body during the pre-season, so caution must be taken during this training cycle to avoid letting your "eyes be bigger than your stomach." Because energy expenditure is greater as a result of more sports-specific, intense training and competitions, your first inclination may be to eat and keep eating. However, it is important to stay in continual check with your body and listen to the hunger and satiety cues. If you did indeed teach your body to become more metabolically efficient to use more of your internal fat stores as energy and preserve your carbohydrate stores during higher-intensity exercise, you will likely not feel as hungry after a training session and thus will not have to replenish as many carbohydrate stores. Of course, there are many factors involved, including your body's aerobic fitness level and current nutrition program; unfortunately, one size doesn't fit all.

It is still important to have a well-balanced feeding before training so that your body is in a well-fed and hydrated state. However, if it is a high-quality training session, extra carbohydrates may be needed. Be sure to keep sources of lean protein and healthy fat in the feeding before competition in order to maintain good blood sugar and insulin levels and thus improve your body's ability to use fat as fuel.

Fluid

Hydration status is bound to change as a result of changing environments and increased heat production in the body from more intense training and competition; with this comes the need for you to listen to your body even more. The range of drinking 3–8 ounces every 15–20 minutes during training can still apply, and it is even more important during this training cycle to drink based on thirst instead of drinking ahead of your thirst. This helps you remain in fluid balance without risking the change of developing hyponatremia, which can be caused by fluid overload. More information about hyponatremia is presented in Chapter 6.

Carbohydrate

Keeping in mind the concept of metabolic efficiency and not overfeeding the body with a huge amount of carbohydrate without lean protein and healthy fats, it is important to realize that your body likely needs supplemental carbohydrates with higher-intensity or longer-duration training. However, it does not need as many extra carbohydrates as you think if you have indeed taught your body to utilize more of its internal fat stores for energy during training. That said, following the "less is more" idea with carbohydrates is a good plan of action during training. In brief, start at the lower end of carbohydrate recommendations per hour and increase as needed based on your energy levels. Although the recommendations of grams of carbohydrate to consume per hour do not fall below 30, many metabolically efficient athletes have sustained good intense efforts of 2–3 hours on 10–20 grams (40–80 calories) of carbohydrate per hour. Beginning in a lower range does not hurt your performance because you can always add more during your training session. However, starting too high at first can increase your risk of GI distress.

Protein

A great deal of protein is not needed during most training sessions. Because the body's energy needs are satisfied mostly from internal stores of carbohydrate and fat, it is not necessary to configure a large amount of protein into the nutrition plan during training or competition. A small amount (3–10 grams per hour), as mentioned in the discussion of the pre-season cycle, can be added, but it does not constitute a major portion of your energy intake.

Fat

Athletes who compete in ultra-endurance (more than 12 hours) events and those who train for long durations and miss meals because of training are typically the groups of athletes who need to eat more fat during training or competition. Ultra-endurance athletes require more fat during this training cycle because of the higher energy expenditure from longer training. These athletes can usually not satisfy all of their energy needs from eating carbohydrates alone. Food choices greatly depend on the athlete's taste preferences and digestive system, and can range from trail mix, to liquid sources of calories with fat, to peanut butter and jelly (or honey) sandwiches. As mentioned previously, the type of fat that is consumed is important. Fat from monounsaturated and polyunsaturated sources is recommended.

Sodium

Now that the training load has increased, maintaining fluid balance becomes much more important. Because of the positive role that sodium plays in improving fluid balance, research indicates the quantity of sodium that most athletes should consume per hour. This amount, 500–700 milligrams per liter of fluid consumed, may or may not meet the needs of some athletes. For those who have high sweat rates or have challenges staying hydrated, more sodium per hour may be required. Additionally, because sodium is also important for conducting nerve transmission and muscle contraction, and because some athletes may be performing more explosive training that requires the facilitation of better muscle functioning, adding more sodium to the hourly nutrition plan can be beneficial. Also, weight-class athletes may require more sodium following the weigh-in in order to rehydrate. In my work with athletes, I begin at 800 milligrams per hour and increase based on individual needs.

FUELTIP

Following a low-sodium daily diet is important from a health perspective and should be the norm for most athletes. Using a higher-sodium load, either immediately before, as described previously, or during exercise, is meant to sustain physiological functioning for athletes to improve performance. Using this high amount of sodium on a regular basis outside of training sessions or competitions is not recommended.

After Training

This is certainly the time of the training cycle when paying particular attention to nutrition in the post-training or post-competition timeframe is of extreme importance. Current research states that it is important for athletes to consume nutrients within 30–60 minutes following quality training because this is when insulin sensitivity is at its highest and muscles are more apt to "accept" nutrients. Even though this is absolutely the case, I prefer to use a "1- to 15-minute rule" with most athletes to ensure that the nutrients are consumed before the 60 minutes are up.

Schedules or traveling to and from workouts often impair the ability for some athletes to start their refueling and rehydration plan immediately after training; thus it is important to plan ahead. If you know you will not be able to have an adequate snack or meal within this hour time frame, bring a ready-to-drink smoothie, a sandwich, or a pre-packaged post-workout powder to have.

However, it is important to mention the concept of microcycle nutrition periodization. Athletes have both quality and non-quality training sessions throughout the week. Based on the physical objectives for each workout, post-workout nutrition could be of utmost importance or not as important. Looking at your training on a daily basis and correlating your nutrition to support your energy expenditure ensures that you are putting the right amount of food in your body when it needs it the most without overfeeding your body when the workout was simply not intense enough or long enough in duration to support eating a high amount of food. For example, on high-intensity or longer-duration (greater than 2 hours) training days, it may be more beneficial to eat more calories by including an immediate post-workout feeding because nutrient and fluid stores are compromised by the higher physical stress. However, on recovery or aerobic-based training days (no intensity or less than 2 hours), scheduling your training to end before meal or snack time more than supports your body's nutrient needs. It is important to separate your post-workout nutrition plan into this nutrition microcycle mind-set so that you always receive the correct amount of nutrients when needed and are not overfeeding your body on days when your energy expenditure is low.

Fluid

Just as during the pre-season, after training or competition, fluid recommendations are extremely important to follow. Aim to drink 24 ounces of fluid for every pound that you lose during training, but remember, preventing a significant loss of body weight from fluid should be your main goal. Thus be sure to pre-hydrate and follow adequate hydration guidelines during training or competition to minimize the amount that you have to drink afterward.

Carbohydrate

Now may be the time to adhere to the current research recommendations of consuming 1.0–1.2 grams of carbohydrate per kilogram of body weight. For most athletes weighing between 50–100 kilograms (110–220 pounds), this means eating about 200–480 calories from carbohydrate.

FUELTIP

Although this is purely anecdotal information, I have noticed that athletes who have taught their bodies to become more metabolically efficient in the pre-season do not require as many carbohydrates in the post-training or competition window. This is because they use more fat for energy during training and rely less on carbohydrate stores. Less carbohydrates used means less carbohydrates that are needed to be replenished. Thus, for these athletes, eating a large amount of carbohydrate after a training session or competition may simply not be needed.

Protein

It is very important to consume protein after training. Although a specific ratio or percentage has not been justified by research, absolute amounts have been indicated. Aim for consuming 10–25 grams of protein in the post-workout window. The "more is better" approach does not hold true in this case.

Fat

As you learned in the pre-season post-workout nutrition recommendations, fat competes with carbohydrate absorption; thus consuming a good amount of fat in the 1- to 60-minute window is not necessary. Similar to before, having a little fat with other protein-rich foods is fine as long as it is kept to a minimum. Ideally, the fat would be comprised of mono- or polyunsaturates and very little saturated and trans fats. This helps control the inflammatory response (discussed in Chapter 6).

> **FUELTIP**
>
> If you have been following the metabolic efficiency concept throughout this chapter, you may be putting some things together that puzzle you. Specifically, if you teach your body to use more fat during a session and thus need fewer carbohydrates afterward, as noted in the last FuelTip, does it make sense to eat more fat in the post-workout window? Interestingly, there are data to show that intramuscular triglycerides (stored fat) are used during exercise. I know that may not be new information, but the important take-home message is that there is no conclusive research on whether or not you have to consume a good amount of fat in the post-workout window to replenish what is used. At this time, I do not recommend including much fat in the 1- to 60-minute window until there is more conclusive evidence to show its benefit.

Sodium

Because of the fluid balance properties of sodium and its ability to improve hydration status after training and competition, it is recommended to consume at least 500 milligrams of sodium in the 1- to 60-minute post-workout or competition window. This can be done through drinks, food, or electrolyte capsules/fluids based on your individual taste preferences.

Here is an example to help you develop a post-workout nutrition plan to use during this training cycle. This is based on a male athlete who is 5'10" tall and weighs 170 pounds (77.3 kilograms).

Step 1: Figure carbohydrate requirements.

- I use the upper recommendation of 1.2 grams of carbohydrate per kilogram of body weight. (Remember to adjust according to your own training level.)

  1.2 grams of carbohydrate × 77.3 kilograms of body weight = 93 grams

- Convert grams to calories.

  93 grams of carbohydrate × 4 calories per gram of carbohydrate = 372 calories

Step 2: Figure protein requirements

- I use 10 grams of protein in this example.

10 grams of protein × 4 calories per gram of
protein = 40 calories

This athlete should eat a total of 412 calories within 15 minutes of finishing his training session. If you are an athlete who just cannot stomach food post-workout, don't worry. Your best bet to get the calories in your body is to reach for a liquid source, such as a skim milk–based fruit smoothie or a pre-formulated post-workout nutrition beverage.

Nutrition for the Off-Season

The off-season can mean different things, depending on the athlete and the sport. For some athletes, this time of the training year brings a complete break from training; others may engage in regular exercise without structure. Regardless, these are the normal nutritional goals that can be implemented during this cycle:

1. Managing emotions in order to manage calorie intake. Emotional eating patterns are often higher during the off-season because training is lower and the athlete has more time during the day to think about food.

2. Identifying the necessary nutritional shift needed to support a lower energy expenditure. "Eating to train" should not be the mantra that athletes follow during this cycle because, as long as an athlete is in fact in an off-season, energy expenditure is not high; thus eating to prepare for a training session should not be the psychological focus. Instead, eating to support health should be the goal during exercise sessions.

3. Discontinuing the use of sports nutrition supplements. The extra calories from these types of products are simply not needed during this cycle. Athletes should be encouraged to supply their daily calorie needs from whole foods rather than

sports nutrition products such as energy bars, gels, drinks, and powders.

4. Preventing body weight and fat gain. If the off-season lasts less than 3 weeks, there is no point in attempting to lose significant body weight. Behavior change research shows that the minimum time to develop a behavior change is 3 weeks. Personally, I believe that, in "real-life" settings, it is more like months or years, but the take-home message is that preventing weight and body fat gain should be the main goal during any off-season lasting 1–21 days.

This is normally the time of the year when most nutritional mistakes are made because of the abrupt change in energy expenditure coming off of the competition season. The off-season typically includes a significant reduction in both volume and intensity because it is the time when most athletes take a physical and mental break from training and competition. Because of this quick change from season to season, it is difficult for many athletes to manage their nutrition to support their reduction in overall exercise. Thus, unnecessary weight gain is the normal response.

FUELTIP

Some athletes compete at a lower than normal body weight during the competition cycle; thus they have to get their body weight back to normal during the off-season. This necessary weight gain should be encouraged for health purposes.

The common physical goals that athletes normally have during this time of the year are to have fun trying new exercise modes without the added pressure of exercising on a schedule, rehabilitating nagging injuries, and possibly even taking a short, extended break from activity altogether. It is therefore important to note the association between weight gain and the decrease in energy expenditure.

Quantitative Recommendations

Daily carbohydrate intake should range from 3–4 g/kg during this cycle. The amount is fairly low, once again, because of the physical goals associated with this cycle and the lower overall energy expenditure. It is most beneficial to acquire the majority of carbohydrates during this cycle through fruits and vegetables while keeping whole grains at minimal amounts.

Protein intake should range from 1.5–2.3 g/kg. For most athletes, I recommend consuming toward the higher range for improving satiety, stabilizing the hunger response throughout the day, and contributing to positive protein stores if strength training is a part of the exercise program.

Fat intake should range from 1.0–1.2 g/kg. Fat is still important to include in the daily nutrition program, even though energy expenditure is not high. More mono- and polyunsaturated fat should be the main focus, specifically omega-3 sources. Saturated and trans fats should be minimized to the lowest level possible.

Fluid

During this time of the year, it is best to establish your fluid balance instinct again without adhering to specific hydration guidelines. Focus on eating high water-containing foods, such as fruits and vegetables, throughout the day and listen to your body's cues regarding hydration balance. Note your thirst response and your color and frequency of urine to assess if you should hydrate more or not. A little subjectivity can go a long way during this cycle in teaching you how to listen to your body once again, which is of extreme importance before heading into your pre-season.

Table 3.4
Summary of Daily Nutrition Needs during the Off-Season Mesocycle

Training Cycle	CHO	PRO	FAT
Off-season	3–4 g/kg	1.5–2.3 g/kg	1.0–1.2 g/kg

Qualitative Recommendations: The FuelTarget™

Because this is the off-season and energy expenditure is lower compared to that in the competition season, it is easy to recommend the FuelTarget™ Zone 1 and possibly Zone 2 if you are exercising for more than a couple of hours per day (in one or more disciplines, such as cardiovascular and strength training). Focusing your daily nutrition plan on mostly lean protein, healthy fats, fruits and vegetables, and whole grains with minimal misses helps you balance your energy intake with your energy expenditure. Combining these foods together helps manage your blood sugar more successfully so that you stay fuller longer, which helps prevent unnecessary body weight and fat gain.

FUELTIP

Food serves many different purposes for athletes. It is obviously essential to sustain life, but food should also be fun. Life is way too short not to enjoy what you are putting in your body. Of course, there are times when you must eat certain foods to gain the maximum benefit from their nutrients, but don't be a slave to your food choices. This training cycle is ideal for changing it up a bit and moving outside of your comfort zone in choosing different foods. Mix it up a little by trying new ethnic foods, different food preparation methods, and exotic fruits and vegetables.

THE PERIODIZATION PLATES™

If you refer back to Figure 3.4, showing the Periodization Plates™, the shift of macronutrients supports the FuelTarget™ Zones 1 and 2. The majority of your plate should include fruits and vegetables, with lean protein and healthy fats rounding out the last major area on the plate. Whole grains, if you choose to eat them, should be minimized at all meals and snacks.

FUELTIP

Rotate through different foods and menus in order to get more overall variety and balance in your eating plan. Remember that now is the time to introduce more opportunities for variety because you will likely become a creature of habit as you enter your competition season. Did you know that the average American only eats approximately 50 different foods in a lifetime compared to people in other societies who eat well over 100 different foods? The more variety you have in your eating program, the better the balance of nutrients you will get and the healthier you will be, not to mention the performance benefits you will glean from the increased nutrient offerings.

TRAINING NUTRITION FOR THE OFF-SEASON

Before Exercise

If you are not following a structured training program, there is no need to "eat to train." Similar to the early pre-season meal before a workout, the main goal is to stabilize blood sugar by eating a macronutrient-balanced snack or small meal with adequate water before the workout. Specific nutrient timing systems are not as important if you are simply going to exercise for up to 2 hours without much structure or intensity.

Carbohydrates, Protein, Fat, and Sodium

The most important nutrition message regarding all of these nutrients is that a specific nutrient timing system is not much of a factor in the window before exercise if it lacks structure. Simply eat a macronutrient-balanced snack or small meal 1–2 hours before your workout, just enough to supply your body with the nutrients needed to stabilize blood sugar, and you will be fine during your exercise session.

During Exercise

For most exercise training in the off-season, the only nutrient that needs to be consumed is water—and certainly no sports nutrition products. They are simply not needed if you are not trying to make strength, power, force, or endurance gains. Therefore, focus on drinking water when you feel that your body needs it (developing your instinctual assessment to hydration as stated previously) and do not overfeed yourself with other calorie-containing nutrients.

After Exercise

It may be tempting to revert back to your post-workout nutrition practices of the competition season, but doing so in this cycle adds unwanted pounds and body fat to your body. The best thing to do after exercising is to repeat the snack or small meal that you had before exercise. It doesn't have to be the same exact food combinations, but ensuring that you have lean protein, a bit of healthy fat, carbohydrates from fruits and vegetables, and water provides your body with the nutrients that may have been lost during exercise. Although it is best to try to eat within the hour following exercise, it is not as imperative for recovery as it was during the last training cycle. If there is not glycogen-depleting exercise performed during this cycle, you simply do not have to worry about eating to improve recovery. Focus on combining the right foods rather than using sports nutrition products.

PUTTING NUTRITION PERIODIZATION TO THE TEST

I often get asked by coaches and athletes if nutrition periodization really works. I have collected body composition data on some athletes with whom I have worked. It shows positive athlete improvement by using the principles of nutrition periodization that accomplish their main purpose of manipulating body weight and composition.

Although the following information is purely anecdotal, based on my work with athletes in and out of competition, it will hopefully provide you with some quantitative information to prove that the concepts you have read about are worth adopting into your yearly training periodization plan. Remember, nutrition should support your physical training so that you are able to induce positive physiological adaptations and continually compete at an optimal level of performance.

These tables contain weight and body composition data obtained from the Bod Pod, which is a body composition measuring device.

These data on body composition were from a female Division I collegiate diver who was trying to lose weight (Table 3.5). As you can see, she was able to decrease her body weight by 1.1 pounds and her body fat by 2.5%, and increase her lean body weight by 2.5 pounds in 4 months by implementing a periodized approach to her nutrition. Although this may not seem like a huge gain, keep in mind that this was during her competition season, so her progress was right on track to avoid a negative impact on her performance as a result of weight and body fat loss.

Table 3.5
Body Composition Trend for a Collegiate Female Diver

	Weight (lbs)	Body Fat %	LBW (lbs)
Sep	131.7	20.6	104.5
Nov	133.9	19.9	107.3
Dec	131.6	18.5	107.3
Jan	130.6	18.1	107

This example of a female Division I collegiate sprint track athlete was one of my most successful athlete stories by far (Table 3.6); as you can see, she reduced her body weight by 6.8 pounds and her body fat by 6.9%, and increased her lean body weight by 4.5 pounds in 5 months through nutrition periodization. Her performance improved more than it ever had in the past. She was extremely motivated and executed her nutrition periodization plan to a tee.

Table 3.6
Body Composition Trend for a Collegiate Female Sprinter

	Weight (lbs)	Body Fat %	LBW (lbs)
Sep	153.8	15.7	129.6
Oct	152.2	12.5	133.1
Nov	150.7	11.5	133.3
Dec	150.8	12	132.7
Mar	147	8.8	134.1

These data from a female Division I collegiate gymnast provide another example of an athlete being successful when the energy is applied to making a nutritional and behavioral change (Table 3.7). She reduced her body weight by 5.6 pounds and her body fat by 5.6% and increased her lean body weight by 1.9 pounds in 5 months. This amount of change significantly reduces the chance of injury while competing.

Table 3.7
Body Composition Trend for a Collegiate Female Gymnast

	Weight (lbs)	Body Fat %	LBW (lbs)
Aug	119.5	22	93.3
Oct	117.6	19	95.2
Nov	117	19.4	94.3
Dec	115.8	18.1	94.9
Jan	113.9	16.4	95.2

This is an example of a male Division I collegiate cross-country runner who wanted to lose weight in order to run faster (Table 3.8). The nutrition intervention was made during his off-season from fall cross-country to winter indoor track; as you can see, he lost 3.4 pounds and 3.5% body fat and increased his lean body weight by 1.9 pounds by following a periodized nutrition plan.

Table 3.8
Body Composition Trend for a Collegiate Male Cross-Country Runner

	Weight (lbs)	Body Fat %	LBW (lbs)
Nov	146.5	10.7	130.8
Dec	144.5	9.6	130.4
Jan	143.1	7.2	132.7

As much as I like to emphasize the successes achieved by following the principles of nutrition periodization, it is also important for me to discuss the setbacks. The athlete depicted in Table 3.9 was a male Division I collegiate swimmer who constantly had trouble with his body weight and composition during his tapers. As the first two columns increase and the last decreases, the athlete transitions into a week-long taper before an important competition. His events were never as good as in training because of this body weight and fat increase during this week. This is a great example of what forgetting to periodize your nutrition can do. Almost universal is the taper training principles of reduced volume with the maintenance of intensity. If this holds true in your sport, remember that you do not have to eat the same amount of food during your taper.

Table 3.9
Body Composition Trend for a Collegiate Male Swimmer

	Weight (lbs)	Body Fat %	LBW (lbs)
Sep	165	8.2	151.7
Dec	165.4	10.3	148.4
Jan	167.1	8.2	153.4
Mar	168.3	11.9	148.3

Regardless of which sport you participate in, if you do not alter your eating plan, specifically the quantity of food you eat, during your taper, you are very likely to gain weight, which may lead to a decrease in your performance. As you will learn in the next chapter, simply changing your nutritional habits on a drop of a dime is unrealistic for most athletes because it is a change of habit. I will give you good strategies that you can use to help with this.

SUMMARY

Having a periodized nutrition plan year-round to support your health and training cycles improves your performance. It doesn't matter if you are in the highest-intensity training cycle or your off-season. The important point is that you must have a well-planned nutrition program that is aligned with your annual training plan and that meets your changing energy expenditure needs during each of your yearly periodization cycles.

Don't underestimate the power of nutrition. You are an expert on how your body works and functions, so become more in tune with your specific nutrition needs and use the information presented here to develop an individualized eating program tailored to your health and training. Remember, eat to train, don't train to eat!

4

Successful Weight Management

If there is one thing that has been reinforced to me since writing the first edition of this book, it is that, at some point throughout their sport career, athletes want to change the way they look, feel, and perform. Although that may not seem like a groundbreaking statement, what is interesting is that changing body weight and/or body composition is consistent among young and old, men and women, and recreational and elite athletes. It can be for the improvement of health, performance enhancement, aesthetics, or all three. However, the majority of athletes with whom I have come in contact want to use weight and body fat loss as a performance improvement strategy as a primary goal, while using the benefits of weight loss to affect their health positively. These are the athletes who commonly state that losing weight helps them be stronger or faster. The trend has mostly been toward body weight or fat reduction, although some athletes want the opposite. No matter what your body weight or composition goals are, there are methods and appropriate timing strategies to employ in your training year to do this so that you do not jeopardize your performance or immune function.

Another important point is the difference between weight loss and fat loss. Often, they go hand in hand, but my focus is not always on reducing the number on the scale. A reduction of body fat and an increase in lean muscle mass are advantageous for health and performance reasons for most athletes unless they are in a weight-cutting phase where absolute pounds matter in order to compete.

I don't believe in "diets." In fact, I don't even care to use that word in a normal conversation. There are two main reasons for this. The first is that the word "diet" carries a negative connotation. Eating should be fun. It should be an enjoyable part of your life and one that you look forward to. The second is that you are an athlete, and because you follow a training program, you should follow an eating program. It doesn't matter if you are recreationally active or an elite athlete. As you learned in the previous chapter, your eating program should support your training program. Diets come and go and are typically extremely unrealistic and unsuccessful. Following an eating program is more successful because you adopt it as part of your lifestyle.

Let me qualify some things before we get too far into the nuts and bolts of this chapter. I'm not your typical registered dietitian who discusses the food pyramid, calorie levels, and the like. That information is useful for some populations, but when it comes to the athletic population, I have discovered that you are, well, different. You know this, as do I. Your priorities are different, and your approach to food is much different than non-athletes. I have focused my career on sports nutrition, working with a wide variety of athletes, and I have realized that food can be an obsession similar to working out. Food serves two purposes in your lives: function and reward. Functionally, food provides you with energy to support your training sessions (the "eat to train" mantra). You provide your bodies with calories so that you can successfully have energy for or recover from training sessions. This is what I term "conscious eating." That is, you plan the nutrition before, during, and after training or competition to ensure that your body has the correct amount and quality of foods to support the physical stressors you throw at it.

The reward side of food for you is purely psychological and emotional, or as I term it, "subconscious eating." You may not know it by this term, but you certainly know it when it happens to you. These are the times when you eat, but you are not sure why you are eating. You could be sad, upset, happy, stressed, tired, or bored. Maybe it was a bad day at work, or you didn't hit your training goals for the day, or you didn't get enough sleep the night before. Regardless of the reason, this pattern of eating is the cause of about 95% of the nutrition challenges that I encounter with athletes. Food is typically not the root of the problem. The patterns and habits that steer you to certain foods, and what you do after you identify your "trigger" foods and situations, are the challenges. This is easy to identify in any athlete by simply observing the "why" behind eating patterns. Like most dietitians, I firmly believe in asking an athlete to complete a 3-day food log. However, my unique approach focuses more on the psychological trends rather than the choice of foods. Don't get me wrong—there are many athletes who simply need a "nutrition makeover" that provides them with better choices of foods to eat. However, this is the easy fix. Eventually, these athletes have to face the psychological and emotional challenges of why they are eating what they are eating. It happens to all of you sometime during your journey through sport. For the majority of athletes, I recommend keeping track of what, when, and why you eat during this food logging cycle. I don't care much for using scales, measuring cups, or spoons. You know if you overeat and certainly don't need these measuring devices to reinforce it. This is not the issue at hand. Many athletes do not believe me at first when I say that the quantity and quality of food that you eat is not your biggest challenge—it is actually the easy part. The true challenge is to determine why you are eating certain foods at certain times. What are your emotional triggers that predispose you to certain types and amounts of food? These are your obstacles for weight and body fat loss (and gain in some athletes). This is your crutch that has been supporting your unsuccessful attempts to change the way your body looks, feels, and performs. Control your mind, and you control your body.

A DIFFERENT APPROACH

Most sports nutrition books that discuss weight management strategies only discuss the calories-in versus calories-out (technically known as the energy balance equation). Although this can be a valuable educational tool, many athletes fail to realize that manipulating body weight for health, performance, or aesthetics is never as easy as counting calories, at least in the long term. Throughout this chapter, I present three very different steps for manipulating body weight and composition: (1) instinctual, (2) qualitative, and (3) quantitative, in the order of importance. For the hundreds of athletes with whom I have worked, counting calories has never enabled them to succeed long term with their weight/body composition goals. Thus, it is important to understand and embrace the first two steps prior to using the third step—counting calories. Remember, manipulating body weight and composition is about the emotions, not about the calories.

BEHAVIOR CHANGE

Besides the psychological and emotional influences of eating, habit formation is a close second when it comes to providing you with more obstacles in your quest for weight loss. Habits can be formed easily and quickly, whereas changing or breaking them could take weeks, months, or even years. You may already know that it takes at least 21 days to change a behavior. You are the lucky one if that is the case for you! In my experience, most athletes require 2–8 months simply to change a behavior and even longer to reinforce it into a maintenance phase.

Before I became a sport dietitian, I worked extensively in the wellness field and specialized in behavior change and goal setting. These were valuable years for my professional development because I was able to learn and implement different strategies of helping people make behavior changes. I gained the knowledge of what it truly takes to break and reform habits, and I had the most success by using the psychological theory, the Stages of Change Model (SCM), that has existed since the late 1970s and early 1980s. James Prochaska and Carlo DiClemente developed the SCM at the University of Rhode Island while studying how smokers tried to end their addiction. The rationale behind this model is that behavior change involves a progression through many steps before the behavior is fully changed. These steps do not have a timeline; many athletes progress at their own rate and should be allowed to do so without outside influence.

This is not an extensive explanation of this theory—there are books that do this much better—but it is important to understand the basics of each stage so that you can have a better understanding of how to use it, how to identify the starting point for your weight loss goals, and how to progress from stage to stage. The stages are the following:

Precontemplation:	In this stage, you do not acknowledge that there is a problem behavior to change, and you do not think seriously about changing. You are not interested in receiving any assistance from anyone, and you defend your habit by not thinking that it is a problem. You may be 20 pounds overweight and not realize that it is a problem yet, and when someone, perhaps a close friend or family member, tries to tell you, you adamantly deny it. Simply put, you just don't see yourself as having a problem yet.
Contemplation:	In this stage, you actually spend time thinking about changing your habit, but you don't act on it. It is purely a cognitive stage where thinking about it is the extent of your progression. This stage is like riding a teeter-totter. You go up and

	down weighing the pros and cons of changing but never progress further. You are more open to receiving information about changing your habit and use educational methods to reflect on your thoughts and feelings of making the change. You accept the handouts I give you about the benefits of losing 20 pounds and think about them, but you just won't act yet.
Preparation:	In this stage, you are committed to making a change, and you have fully embraced beginning the actual process by seeking out information to help you change your behavior. Small steps toward attaining your goal are the focus. For example, it could be identifying your meal timing and patterns throughout the day; if stress, boredom, or emotions trigger eating higher-fat foods or higher quantities; or you begin reading my handouts and other educational information.
Action:	In this stage, you believe in yourself and in the ability to change your behavior, lose weight, and be successful. Maybe it is shopping for healthier foods, not eating dessert, choosing not to eat out any longer, or meeting with a registered dietitian who specializes in sports nutrition. The important thing is that you are actively involved in the change. Because this is the stage where you rely more on your willpower, it can be volatile because the risk for relapse is high. However, you form solutions to possible obstacles that you face, both from yourself and from

your friends and family. Short-term rewards are used by some, with great success. Just be sure that you are not using food as a reward for your great progress. Try something else, such as a new pair of shoes or another piece of clothing, a new watch, or something that is a tangible and healthy reward. The last thing to note about this stage is that you are willing to seek support from others, which can help prevent relapse. Develop a positive support system—those who you can depend on in times of trouble—and use them. It will assist you tremendously in progressing to the final stage.

Maintenance:　The action stage may or may not take you a while to complete, but once you get to this stage, you often have the skills to stay here. Short bouts of relapse may happen, as I discuss, but for the most part, you have done the work to change your habit, and now you will maintain it. This stage involves being able to avoid successfully any temptations that get thrown your way to return you to your habit. I see this quite frequently with athletes after they have lost weight and then a holiday, birthday, or other special occasion sneaks up on them. These are merely tests—ones that knock on your door and continue to do so until you open it and do something about them. One characteristic of this stage is the ability to anticipate situations that may cause a relapse and have already proven coping strategies ready and waiting.

In the preceding example, you know you will be attending a social engagement where there will be unhealthy food choices that you do not prefer to eat because you have worked so hard to lose your weight and develop new habits. By eating something beforehand and merely drinking water during the gathering, or having small portions if you have to eat something because of social pressure, you will be able to make it through successfully without worries. You may still have thoughts of returning to your old behavior every so often, but you resist these temptations and keep focused on your new changes.

Relapse

Although relapse is not a defined stage of progression in the SCM, it is important to mention because it is absolutely natural to regress. Remember, this is a behavior change and is a completely normal part of making changes. Some athletes experience a relapse; others encounter quite a few. Relapse can certainly be discouraging and take a bite out of your self-confidence, but it is important to understand that the SCM considers this to be part of your journey of change. In fact, most athletes cycle through the five stages several times before achieving a successful lifestyle change. Don't expect this to happen overnight or even within a few months. It takes work on your part, but, again, expect relapse. If you approach this behavior change with the idea that there will be hurdles and obstacles that prevent you from being successful at times, you are more apt to allow these to come and go without sending you into a downward spiral where you discontinue your progression. If you slip on occasion, remember, you are not a bad person, and you have not failed. You are merely encountering the natural progression of changing a behavior. If something does happen, take the opportunity to analyze why. Were you served your absolute favorite dessert in the world at the social gathering and just could not say no? Use this as an opportunity to develop different coping strategies.

One thing to note about relapse is that, when it happens, be sure to not regress to the precontemplation or contemplation stages. It is extremely important to restart your process at the preparation, action, or, even better, the maintenance stage.

Consider this example as more explanation. Your goal is to lose 20 pounds for performance reasons. You know you want to start, but you just may not be ready yet. If I tell you that you have to lose this weight and seeing me once a week is mandatory, chances are that you will still not do it. Remember, you cannot force a change in behavior. You must want to progress through the steps rather than being told to do so. Not only do you have to decide when it is the right time to seek the change, but it is up to you to determine how quickly or slowly you progress from stage to stage. This decision must come from within. The most important thing to remember is that you should not lose the weight for anyone except for yourself. I know this may be tough if a coach is encouraging you or your sport mandates a specific weight to compete, but your success rate will be less if you do it for the wrong reasons.

My fairly simple steps that are presented throughout this chapter make change less of a burden because of the simplicity, which means that you will have a higher success rate—not only at changing behavior but also at adopting it into your lifestyle. Believe me, I have helped hundreds of athletes accomplish weight loss goals, and, even though every athlete and every weight loss strategy is different, what I have learned is that if you do not want to do it for yourself, you will not succeed in the long term.

Losing weight or decreasing body fat is easy when you look at it on paper. I mean, how hard could it be to balance what goes in your body with what is going out? Eat less and exercise more, and you will be a slimmer you. Unfortunately, it is not that easy, as you have likely experienced if you have ever tried to lose weight and actually maintain it for more than a year. This length of time is important because there has been much research done on individuals who lose weight and on their success rate at regular intervals. What most research has shown is that the quick-fix, "too good to be true" diets produce weight loss in the initial stages, but after one year, most individuals return to their original weight, and in some cases, actually tack on another 5–15 pounds. This typically happens because the "diet" that is followed is so unrealistic to maintain that it is like a time bomb, programmed to go off after only a short time. It's inevitable and, unfortunately, typically sends the person into a downward spiral of what I call "diet hopping." These are the athletes who, when I am talking to them, describe themselves as having tried every diet known to man, yet they are still trying to lose weight. If this sounds like you, keep reading. I think you will be both intrigued and pleasantly surprised by my simple, no-gimmick, tried and true, scientifically-based, non-calorie counting approach to weight loss.

This is a topic that I take very seriously and one that I have great success at with athletes as long as two "conditions" are met prior to starting. First, you have to be willing to forget any of the diet quick-fixes you have ever done; second, you must promise both you and me that you will not revert to those old habits while you are embarking on using my methods. The second is a bit more difficult, but if you do it, you will succeed. You must trust me and my methods. You may not know me other than what you have read, but if you can instill this trust in me, you will be successful. I have had the most success with athletes who adopt my weight loss principles as a lifestyle change, not a temporary solution. These are the athletes who not only seem to reap the health benefits, but also the performance-enhancing gains that accompany better health.

I have many examples of the athletes with whom I have worked in the past, but one athlete in particular exemplifies what it means to provide unconditional trust, even though her doubts were high. This athlete was a female collegiate track athlete, a sprinter. She came to me with the goal of losing weight, but most important, losing body fat. Over a period of five months, I was able to help her lose almost 7 pounds and almost 7% body fat. She is only one of many athletes with whom I have had the pleasure of

seeing positive results, and I attribute her success to two things:
(1) she wanted to make changes to become a better athlete; and
(2) she trusted me unconditionally, and even though she was a bit
weary in the beginning, she maintained her trust because she not
only felt and looked better, but she was also running faster and
with more energy. I should note that she was hesitant with me at
first because I did not prescribe calories to her. We discussed her
emotional cues to eating, and I implemented my very simple qualitative method, which allowed her greater flexibility and less stress
than counting calories.

As I am sure you know, weight loss success is not all glam-
orous and happy. The preceding example happens more often
than not when I work with athletes, but there are a few that just
do not find success with my, or any other, methods of weight
loss. I worked with a female swimmer on a weight-loss program,
and she actually progressed backwards in five months. She
gained body weight, body fat, and lost lean muscle mass. Even
though I had the luxury of seeing her weekly (and daily sometimes), we still were not having the results we wanted. After
many discussions with the athlete and taking food completely out
of the conversations (remember, weight loss has more to do with
psychology for most athletes), we both realized that she was not
at the proper stage of change that would provide her with a positive start to initiating a change. It just wasn't the right time, nor
were her motivations in line with being successful. It was like a
weight was lifted off of her shoulders when we both came to this
conclusion, and after even more meetings, we discovered that she
was receiving too many outside pressures for losing weight,
which had made her rebel, shut down, and not want to lose
weight for herself. She knew she needed to do it, but the extrinsic
pressures were outweighing her intrinsic motivators. She did not
want to do it for herself, and that is the most important piece of
this body-changing, weight-loss puzzle. You must want to do it
for yourself—first and foremost. It's a long journey and one on
which you truly find out who your biggest supporters are versus
those pressuring you to make the change. Typically, you don't

hear from the latter, and if you do, the conversation is always centered quantitatively on how much weight you have lost rather than on how you are doing, feeling, and whether you need anything to help you accomplish your goals.

SUPPORT SYSTEM

What a great segue way to discuss an extremely important component of your success: your support system. This is commonly overlooked in most athletes embarking on the weight-loss journey, but a team approach has been scientifically proven to be the best method of success, not only in losing weight but in maintaining it. It may sound like an easy concept to grasp. Of course, you have a support system; the commonly chosen one is family and/or friends. The key is that you have a positive support system. There is a significant difference between a support system and a positive support system. The latter is ideal because it is comprised of individuals who have your best interest in mind and who support you by helping you progress through each of the Stages of Change. These people are there for you, no matter what, are never judgmental, and give you that extra "push" when you need it, but in a nonthreatening manner.

The opposite is those who do not understand why you are trying to lose weight, do not adapt their eating habits to assist you in yours, and never have a positive thing to say to you, even when you are succeeding. It is almost as if they want you to fail but do not admit it. This ever-so-important step in your journey should not be overlooked, and you should actually spend some thought-process time selecting your positive support system.

I know you may be asking yourself, "What if these people have to be in my support system because they are family or close friends but I don't want them?" This is a great question and one that you handle by keeping these individuals in the outer circle of your support team. Keep them updated once in a while, but maintain your inner circle with the handful of people who you know always support you no matter what, but who also provide you with the right mix of support and positive motivation.

As you can see, there are many additional factors to discuss pertaining to weight loss that are not centered on calories. Identify your behind-the-scene weight-loss challenges and your plan becomes much clearer and easier to implement. The emotional component of eating is a tremendous thorn in your side. Every athlete I have ever met has had what I term "emotional eating demons." There really is nothing special that associates this problem with athletes. The mere facts that you are human beings and that food is both needed and comforting are enough to cause problems in your approach to food.

If you do not embrace true behavior and habit change, you will not be successful in your journey toward weight loss and body fat loss . For most athletes, manipulating body weight and body composition is not about making smarter food choices. It is about changing your mental approach to food.

There are about as many approaches to weight loss as there are training programs. Each one is unique in its own sense. Some are more credible and can be sustained long term; others promise such fast results, by creating such a low-energy intake, that they are unrealistic to maintain for more than a few weeks at a time. Obviously, the first option is ideal from a health and performance perspective. Athletes are typically not patient. Almost everything you do is based on time, distance, or strength, and now I am asking you to be patient? I realize that changing your body weight is a difficult task in itself because it requires a change of behavior—long-term, sustainable behavior. But I also understand the negative impact of too rapid weight loss on performance. I have seen it firsthand in athletes, and, quite frankly, the majority of athletes who seek fast weight loss usually have compromised immune systems, which leads to a greater incidence of being sick, and not being able to train or simply have enough fuel in their "gas tanks" to finish a workout, let alone recover well. In addition, rapid weight loss dehydrates your body, and I know I do not have to tell you how detrimental that is to performance. In fact, the first few pounds of weight loss can almost always be attributed to a loss of total body water.

As I mentioned previously, there are many ways to approach this change in body weight that you are seeking, and they are dependent on your type of personality. You may be a quantitative or qualitative thinker. Are you a numbers person, or were you not too interested in high school algebra? You may be patient or impatient. Are you known for eating meals in less than five minutes, or do you take the time to put your fork down occasionally? There is not a day that passes when I am not asked by an athlete how many calories or grams of a certain nutrient they should consume. Even though I want nothing more than to provide a simple answer to that question, I cannot do it—because energy expenditure needs associated with different training sessions, along with body weight/composition goals, dictate much of how these questions are answered. You may seek a complex program that provides exact amounts of macro- and micronutrients, but what I have experienced in over 17 years in working with athletes and being an athlete for more than 30 years is that "simple" means "sustainable." For the majority of athletes, a simple eating program, focused on proper nutrient timing and quality of food eaten, elicits the most beneficial results, often sooner than expected. Of course, I encounter the occasional athlete who simply prefers to count calories and work with total grams of carbohydrates, protein, and fat, but this is certainly not the norm. Although I do not prefer this approach for all athletes, I do respect these athletes' thought processes, which is why you will see this strategy included at the end of this chapter.

Personality is the primary trait and dictates the path you take in your weight-loss journey. You can have all the motivation and willpower you want, but if you don't know where you are going and how to get there, it is senseless to proceed. You may actually use a combination of the following methods. That is certainly the ideal model. Imagine the rest of this chapter as your toolbox—a toolbox that I fill with the specific tools to develop, plan, and implement your weight-management program.

Remember, however, as I mentioned earlier, if you are not ready to make a behavior change to manipulate your body weight, it does not matter what type of personality you have or what approach you take. You will be unsuccessful. Progress to the point when you are ready to make the change, to take the leap and trust yourself. It won't be easy at first. No behavior change is. But rest assured that you will be more likely to succeed if you truly are ready for it.

WEIGHT-MANAGEMENT STEPS

Step 1: Become an Instinctual Eater (Again)

I find it interesting that whenever an athlete wants to manipulate (usually lose) body weight and/or body composition, the first thought is to count calories. This normally does not lead to long-term success, and it reinforces being a slave to numbers in the beginning of a behavior change. In fact, the first and most important step when it comes to controlling and manipulating body weight is relearning the body's cues for hunger and satiety. This skill, termed "instinctual eating," is something that you develop at a very young age, but, unfortunately, it is forgotten quickly, as many societal pressures are established throughout the aging continuum, along with confusing marketing messages that are constantly delivered and reinforced to athletes through the media.

Instinctual eating, in simple terms, is a concept that describes feeding the body when it is biologically hungry. Biological hunger can be identified by one of two methods: (1) when physical hunger pangs exist in the stomach and (2) when cognitive functioning and the ability to concentrate and focus decrease. Either of these is your body's way of telling you that it needs food. Instinctual eating is replaced by habitual and emotional eating as you begin to move out of childhood.

Another form of hunger, habitual hunger, is what most athletes experience throughout the day at work and home. A great example of habitual eating is when you use the clock as the marker of telling you it is time to eat. If you eat at certain time intervals throughout the day, not because you are hungry but rather because it may be the standard time for a meal, you are included in this habitual hunger group. You have lost touch with your internal body cues, and they need to be "found" again to incorporate food as an integral part of improving your ability to reconnect with your body's hunger cues.

Lastly, the most popular form of eating for most athletes is emotional eating. It is quite complex, and, although it is never truly mastered, it goes hand in hand with instinctual eating. It should always be the first step for you to identify your emotional connection to food. Emotions are quite powerful and induce both positive and negative thoughts, and with these come incidences of overeating.

The typical emotions that serve as triggers to eating include being sad, depressed, happy, angry, bored, or tired. When one of these triggers is initiated, the resulting outcome is quite often reaching for comfort foods, which are normally high in fat, sugar, salt, or a combination. A healthy relationship with food must be the foremost goal and the first step for any athlete embarking on the goal of manipulating body weight and composition. Without embracing the large role that emotions play, successful weight loss is difficult.

The emotional connection with food definitely requires more discussion because it assists you in moving from a restriction-based nutrition plan, where counting calories is your only focus, to a nonrestriction nutrition plan, where you eat because you identify when and why you are hungry. Table 4.1 depicts the differences between eating, exercise, and progress of weight loss. As can be seen, internalizing how both exercise and nutrition feel is the crucial first step because it sets the mind up for the journey ahead. For example, if you want to lose weight but are always feeling guilty about eating out of fear that it may be the wrong food or that it has too many calories, this is the behavior to work on first. Moving more toward feeling your hunger response and

Table 4.1
Dieting and Non dieting Approaches to Eating, Exercise, and
Progress of Change

Challenge	Diet/Restriction	Non Diet/Restriction
Eating	Do I deserve it? Guilt. Good and bad. Food is the enemy	Am I hungry? Do I want it? Will it be satisfying? Deserve it without guilt.
Exercise	Calories burned. Guilty when missed	How exercise feels.
Progress	Numbers. Aesthetics. What people think	Not primary goal. Self-trust. Internal body cues

eating out of biological hunger is the first goal in your journey. Additionally, I must make note of tracking progress of weight loss. Far too many athletes use the scale as an indicator of weight-loss success (or failure), and this is simply not fair for you to do to yourself. Basing your success on a number that is largely affected by many things that you cannot control—such as hydration status, menstrual cycle patterns, glycogen stores, and bowel movements—makes you a slave to the scale. Because weight can fluctuate up to about 5 pounds in a day, this method of tracking progress does not support your overall goals of weight loss and learning more about your body from the inside out.

Remember that a complete paradigm shift is needed when embarking on the journey of instinctual eating. Quantitative analysis and tracking are not beneficial in the early beginnings, so don't bother with them. I realize this may sound odd, but remember, you are trying to relearn your body, its hunger, its satiety response, and the emotional connection that you have with food. It will not be easy, but it is a mandatory first step. If you skip it and move to the number crunching, you will set yourself up for failure. It is a learning process at first; I normally allow athletes at least 5–7 days as a "break-in" time to begin the behavior change and then another 3–4 weeks to practice the new behavior.

Remember, as described earlier in the Stages of Change section, you always encounter relapse, and that is okay. It is part of changing a behavior, and, because your approach to food is very difficult to change, it takes some time—with much patience. You owe it to yourself to put in this time; this is a lifestyle adaptation and change, not a quick, one-time fix.

As you embark on this journey, goal setting becomes extremely important. Most athletes know this and are keen about setting goals. However, the types of goals formulated in the beginning are often misunderstood, which can lead to more setbacks than successes. The two main goals that are associated with changing a behavior, in this case weight loss, include outcome and process goals. An outcome goal can be defined as the end goal, the ultimate change that you want to make. For example, an outcome goal could be losing 20 pounds. In contrast, a process goal is a stepping stone to help you get to your outcome goal. Unfortunately, many athletes do not realize that it is actually detrimental for a process goal to be a fraction of the total weight loss. For example, if your outcome goal is to lose 20 pounds and you set your process goals to be losing 5 pounds every five weeks, this aids in the restriction mentality, and, quite frankly, can be tied to dieting behavior, which does not withstand the test of time in the success department. Process goals should focus on methods of assisting you to reach your outcome goal, such as learning how to control blood sugar better by combining certain foods together, or timing your nutrient intake to better reflect biological hunger instead of habitual hunger. These examples of process goals yield you much more success in your journey of weight loss.

It is also important not only to acknowledge the small changes that you make, but also celebrate them as successes. Far too often, athletes only focus on the one outcome goal, and, if they do not reach it, they did not succeed. A great example of this is when I worked with a female triathlete once who wanted to lose 15 pounds. She made great progress, but, on the scale, she only lost 12 pounds; to her, because she was so quantitatively based and was not willing to change her paradigm of thinking, she thought of herself as a failure. She did not celebrate the fact that she lost 12 pounds and that she had better health and performance. Because she did not achieve her quantitative outcome goal, she considered her change to be unsuccessful, and she regained the weight once again. Put a plan of action into place that helps you celebrate your successes and positive progress. When you achieve a process goal, reward yourself with items or actions that promote your continued success, not impair it.

Along with this goal-setting exercise, it is important to be a bit selfish and to put yourself at the top of the priority list. Some athletes embark on losing weight for other people; if this is done, it is usually not successful. Once you take responsibility for your goal and becoming more in tune with your body and its hunger signals, you create a better environment to facilitate your weight loss. Keep this process in balance without swaying too much to one side or the other. Hold yourself accountable, but do not become derailed if you encounter what I like to call "speedbumps." These are the little things that take you off your plan temporarily; they include social eating events, stressful days, or missed workouts. Remember, however, as the term "speedbump" implies, you are slowed down, but then once you get over the bump, you gradually return to the same speed again and continue on with your progress.

Fight the urge during this time of relearning your instinctual hunger to use distractions to facilitate weight loss. I have known many athletes who, when biologically hungry, try to mask their hunger so that they eat fewer calories. This can be very problematic. Popular distractions including reading a book, going to the movies, talking on the phone, or exercising—all of which likely facilitate more hunger. For example, if you are trying to avoid your hunger and so you go watch a movie, you may be subconsciously "forced" to have soda and popcorn or candy because you may have done this when you were younger and it is a learned behavior. The take-home message is that you should not be denying your true biological hunger during this step, and distractions should not be part of your repertoire. They cause you to close the hunger door, which negates the overall goal of this first step in relearning your hunger responses. Keep in mind also that the more you deny your hunger, the more intense your food cravings and obsessions become.

Even though I am normally not too supportive of keeping a daily food log, doing so in these initial phases may assist you. However, break free from the common stigma of including how much you eat (calorie counting). That is not necessary at this point and actually works against what you are trying to accomplish. Instead, keep a food log that has three columns: (1) what you eat, (2) when you eat, and (3) why you eat. The last component is the most valuable for you because you will begin to align the reasons that you eat at certain times and choose certain foods. The "why" behind eating is exactly what you are trying to learn; it helps you connect with your biological hunger by realizing when emotional and habitual hunger happen and why.

This process of learning to become an instinctual eater again is not a short-term journey. Instinctual eating exists in your nutrition program each and every day of the year, because it is really the psychological and emotional connection with food that guides your food choices most of the time. Give yourself time in the beginning to learn (and relearn) these processes and continue to develop them month after month. A successful behavior change normally takes more than three weeks to begin, but up to 12 months to become part of your lifestyle.

Step 2: Become a Qualitative Eater

Qualitative Approach

It has been my experience that athletes actually progress and move between both qualitative and quantitative weight-loss methods throughout their weight-loss voyage. Because I have identified the qualitative approach as Step 2, I believe that it belongs before the quantitative, calorie-counting approach to changing body weight and composition. Plus, it serves as a very good assistant in your journey of relearning your body and its instinctual eating patterns.

The qualitative method is centered on three elements: (1) controlling hypoglycemia, (2) incorporating the satiety factor, and (3) utilizing thermogenesis. Throughout your journey, you can use either the FuelTarget™ or Periodization Plates™ concepts (or a combination of both) provided in the previous chapter.

I had the fortunate pleasure of working with an athlete who came to me with weight loss as her primary goal. As with most of the nutrition interventions that I do with athletes, her weight-loss challenges were not primarily food challenges; rather, it was the psychological aspect of her eating that was holding her back. I began by prescribing use of the FuelTarget™ to her because her daily food intake was extremely heavy in the processed carbohydrate category and did not include much macronutrient balance. This, in turn, was causing her to have severe energy lulls during the day and also causing more emotional eating incidents. I knew that this was merely the tip of the iceberg with her, but if we did not address the "low-hanging fruit" first, we would not be able to progress to the next step. The real challenge at hand was not so much choosing the right foods. Believe it or not, that is the easy part. With her, the difficulty was in her emotional tie to certain foods. She understood how to adapt the FuelTarget™ to her life, but it was not easy to execute the plan. Sound familiar? This is what I always refer to as the "easy to say, hard to do" phenomenon. Losing weight sounds easy also, but it isn't. Her emotional obstacles, which we discovered after many discussions (none of which involved eating a specific food), were social gatherings at restaurants and her unselfish behavior.

Many athletes seeking weight loss suffer from these. It is more common than you think. In the case of this athlete, she went to the restaurants that her friends wanted to go to; most often, they were not places where she could follow her FuelTarget™ easily. This caused her to make poor choices and to follow this up with negative self-talk, which is a destructive behavior that people often do in the face of not achieving a goal. I remind you at this time that there are many more positive experiences in our lives than negative ones. It is just human nature to focus and dwell on the negative ones. Try making a list of the good things and the bad things that happen to you in one day. I would be willing to bet there are many more good things than bad. So why do you tend to focus on the bad things? I believe that each athlete has some psychological block that prevents his or her success from being seen. To be more specific, some athletes, at some point in their lives, do not want to be accountable for their actions. I say stand up and deal with these negative experiences. Stare at them eye to eye, and let them be the ones to back down. It is going to happen. You will get down on yourself and doubt your ability to make a positive change. Again, that is part of the behavior change process. It is not a big deal as long as you do not make it out to be one. Accept it and move on. Remember, tomorrow is a new day. The important point is that you adopt this principle: if today you do not succeed as you wanted to with your nutrition plan, let it go and get focused again tomorrow. However, this must be implemented the very next day. If you allow yourself too much time not to be held accountable, it becomes a habit, and a bad one at that.

In my example, as a solution to this restaurant challenge, we decided that it would be beneficial for her to identify three to five restaurants that would support her FuelTarget™ plan. She would then convince her friends to always go to these restaurants so that she regained control. It worked beautifully, and she did not have to feel bad any longer because everyone was happy.

Her second challenge—being unselfish—is extremely common, especially with athletes who want to lose weight because it is often tied to a lower sense of self-confidence because of a higher body weight. This is not about feeling comfortable at your weight. If you are an athlete and you want to lose weight, you will likely not be comfortable with yourself until you attain your goal. That is fine, but remember that, during this time of changing your behavior, you must be selfish. That's correct, I am giving you permission to care about yourself more than others, and that may be difficult at times. Far too often, I see athletes like the one I worked with putting their needs below those of their friends. This is simply not acceptable. If your goal is weight loss, you are the most important person, and you must put your needs above all others. That doesn't mean you should neglect others. It simply means that you must take care of yourself first. By doing this, you embrace the power of behavior change and can fully utilize that energy, as well as your positive support system of friends, family, and teammates, as your assistants in your weight-loss journey. In the case of the athlete I was working with, she was very much a server and wanted to make everyone else happy first. We shifted her thinking and focus to herself first, and she embraced the power that she had to make the right decisions that benefited her. She found it much easier to engage with family and friends, and her self-confidence increased exponentially. Remember, it is okay to put yourself first. You are the only one who truly knows what is in your best interest.

By adopting and implementing these two interventions, this athlete was able to take charge of her life and, more important, attain her weight-loss goals because she was in the driver's seat.

Another great example of adapting to situations is from another female athlete with whom I was working on losing weight. She was traveling via airplane, and before she boarded the plane, she bought a meal that met her personal FuelTarget™. She was very prepared and taking charge of her goals. Although not planning on it, she upgraded to first class, where she was fed a meal en route to her destination. Realizing that she would eat far too much, she opted to discard the food she had bought prior to boarding the plane even though she did not like to waste food. In fact, throwing out food was one of the most difficult things for her to do. She proceeded to eat the meal served to her, and, although she was served foods that did not fall in her FuelTarget™, she did not eat them. This is a fantastic example of having a high level of self-confidence and motivation in pursuit of a personal goal.

As I mentioned in the beginning of my discussion about the qualitative method of weight loss, the three cornerstones associated with it are (1) controlling hypoglycemia, (2) incorporating the satiety factor, and (3) utilizing thermogenesis. Adopting the use of the FuelTarget™ addresses all three of these at almost all times.

Controlling Hypoglycemia

Once your blood sugar dips below a certain level, your craving response increases exponentially. You know what comes next—eat the first thing in sight as long as it is sweet or salty and high in calories! This is the beginning of mindless eating, where you cannot get a hold of the psychological instincts of your body. If you really think about it, a decrease in your blood sugar is a protective mechanism for your brain. Your muscles may not need the nourishment, but your brain does, and it lets you know this extremely fast. You can easily maintain your blood sugar levels throughout the day by following the FuelTarget™ and eating from the inside out. Eating from the inside out is another important concept for you to understand and adopt when using the FuelTarget™, regardless of whether or not you have weight-loss goals. I have experienced too many cases of athletes eating from the outside in and sabotaging themselves.

You know whether you are one of these athletes by performing a simple test. The next time you eat, notice what goes on your plate first. Is it a grain or a lean protein? What goes on second? Is it a fruit or vegetable? It is not uncommon for some athletes to forget a food group completely because of space limitations on a plate. More commonly, it is because their paradigm of thinking is backward. If you focus on eating from the inside of the FuelTarget™ to the outside, you will better prevent hypoglycemia. How? Protein-rich foods combined with fiber-rich foods found in fruits and vegetables have a blood sugar stabilizing effect.

FUELTIP

Fruits and vegetables are great foods; we all know this. But eating one or the other by itself is probably one of the worst things you can do in preventing hypoglycemia. Because of the higher-carbohydrate and lower-protein content of these foods, your blood sugar spikes after about 45–60 minutes, depending on how much you eat, and then drops rapidly and triggers your craving response. This is why it is so important to eat from the inside out of the FuelTarget™ and almost always combine a lean protein/healthy fat with a fruit/vegetable.

Incorporating the Satiety Factor

Satiety, in more simple terms, is basically the feeling of fullness. The more full you feel throughout the day, the more you control your calorie intake and eat less. I may sound like a broken record, but, by following the "eat from the inside out" principle, you will feel fuller longer. It just so happens that lean protein, healthy fat, and the fiber found in fruits and vegetables help you stay fuller longer. You may be wondering why you can't use the fiber in whole grains. You can, but keep in mind that a serving of a whole grain has more calories than a serving of a fruit or vegetable. If your goal is weight loss, acquiring more of your fiber from lower-calorie foods is to your benefit. Physiologically, the body's blood sugar ebbs and flows about every three hours. Thus, what I tell athletes is that if the right type and quantity of foods (eating from the inside out) are put together well, the biological hunger response should not be present for at least three hours throughout the day outside of training session windows.

Utilizing Thermogenesis

Have you ever wondered why some higher-protein diets produce weight loss? Besides the low calorie content of some of them, they are using the biochemical principle that protein has a higher thermic effect of food (TEF) than does carbohydrate or fat. TEF is the term used to describe the metabolic heat loss associated with food intake. Protein has the highest TEF, approximately 20–30%, followed by carbohydrate at approximately 5–10%, followed by fat at approximately 3–5%. These numbers are somewhat insignificant for you to try to use in your daily eating programs; however, the take-home message is that eating a bit more lean protein leads to a higher metabolic heat loss in your body. Remember, heat loss equals calorie loss. I'm not promoting a high-protein diet. Rather, I am reminding you to change your paradigm of thinking by always choosing lean protein and healthy fat as your first menu item so that they are not forgotten. Eat from the inside out, remember?

As discussed in the previous chapter, the FuelTarget™ Zones are a qualitatively based application of the nutrition periodization concept. For athletes seeking weight loss or improved metabolic efficiency, I recommend eating mostly in Zone 1. This includes mostly lean protein, healthy fats, and fruits and vegetables as part of the normal daily eating program. Carbohydrate consumption is worth a short discussion if you navigate your eating in Zone 1. Because whole grains are a minimal component of Zone 1 eating, there are fewer carbohydrates in your daily nutrition plan. Because the brain requires about 130 grams of carbohydrate each day to function properly, it is important to increase your fruit and vegetable intake to accommodate for the carbohydrates not received from whole grains. However, for some athletes, adding more fruits and vegetables may be more difficult than doing an actual competition. Although it takes a few more servings of fruits and vegetables (see Table 4.2) to add up to 130 grams of carbohydrate, it is important to remember that carbohydrates can also be acquired from some lean protein sources, such as beans, nuts, soy products, and milk. Thus, it is easier than you think to fit in all of the necessary carbohydrates that your body needs without many whole grains.

Remember, however, that carbohydrates are not the "bad guy" in your weight-loss goals. Emotional eating, improper timing, and choosing imbalanced macronutrients are the bad guys.

Table 4.2
Servings of Fruit and Vegetables to
Equal 130 Grams of Carbohydrate

9 servings of fruit and 0 vegetables
8 servings of fruit and 2 vegetables
7 servings of fruit and 5 vegetables
6 servings of fruit and 9 vegetables

Many athletes ask why I do not include many whole grains in Zone 1 of the FuelTarget™ or why the Pre-Season Cycle Periodization Plate™ does not include whole grains. The simple answer is that some athletes overindulge in grains so much (eating from the outside in) that I want to ensure that they are consuming the weight-loss-promoting portions of the macronutrients that help in attaining their goal. Additionally, you should very rarely be following a Zone 1 plan if you are engaged in any longer-duration or higher-intensity training. During your weight-loss journey, focus on supplying your brain with the necessary carbohydrates that it needs to function, but not loading up your muscle and liver stores. Save that for later, when your training volume and/or intensity increases.

The combination of eating lean proteins/healthy fats and fruits and vegetables, with a few servings of grains each day, maintains very stable blood sugar levels, prevents hypoglycemia, and keeps you fuller longer. All of which are recipes for success as you are trying to lose weight.

FuelStory #1

I had the pleasure of working with an elite male wrestler in developing a long-term nutrition plan. He was in his mid-twenties and was burned out on his sport because he was tired of constantly having to make weight, and he knew that weight-cutting was not healthy for his body. His walking weight was about 17 pounds higher than his weight class, and even though he admitted that he could cut 10 pounds in 1–2 days if needed, he knew that this drastic a weight-cut significantly impaired his performance. His goal was to get to a walking weight of only 5–7 pounds above his weight class so that it would be easier for him to make weight the week before his competition.

When he first came to me, he had only a couple of weeks before a competition. We both knew we couldn't have a major impact beforehand, so we focused on a few minor changes that were more healthy. I put him in the FuelTarget™ Zone 1 with very limited grains (one serving per day) for one week so that we could determine how his body would respond. One week later, he reported to have lost 3 pounds, and his training was not compromised. He ended up traveling to his competition but did not wrestle because he had a stomach illness. This was probably a blessing in disguise, because, when he came back to see me, he was extremely motivated to construct and execute a nutrition plan that focused more on the long term so that he could prevent the serious weight-cutting practices. We had two months during which he would mostly train, with no competitions. His nutrition recommendations included following Zone 1, drinking to stay hydrated but not overdrinking, and eating frequently.

FUELTIP

Athletes who participate in a sport that has different weight classes, such as wrestling, weightlifting, or boxing, and those with a high degree of aesthetic judging, such as gymnastics, synchronized swimming, or figure skating, do not typically have the luxury of losing weight during their pre-season. Weight-cutting or severe calorie restriction is common in these athletes, and it tends to follow a cyclical pattern surrounding competitions. Although it may not be the preferred method of weight loss, it happens, and it must be taken into account when building an eating program.

Some wrestlers pay very strict attention to the amount of food that they eat, and some count calories. Knowing this, I measured his resting metabolic rate (RMR) so that we would both know and could track where we were starting from a physi-ological standpoint. One of our goals was for him not to eat fewer calories than his RMR; measuring it allowed us to monitor closely his weight-loss progress.

FuelStory #2

A collegiate female sprinter I worked with exemplified the concept of the FuelTarget™ Zone 1, and I termed her my "walking bill-board." The changes that her body went through in the short nine months that we worked together were staggering. I should preface this by stating that she was extremely motivated and had tremendous willpower when her peers would not fully support her new eating program. In the first month that we worked together, she decreased her body weight by only 1.6 pounds but lost 3.2% body fat. From months 2–3, she lost 1.5 pounds and 1% body fat. The most shocking results came from months 4–5, in which she lost 2.2 pounds and 3.2% body fat. Throughout our time together, she lost 6.8 pounds and 6.9% body fat, while increasing her lean muscle mass by 4.5 pounds. Again, this truly exemplified the point that following the FuelTarget™ Zone 1 can work, but it does take motivation and proper execution 95% of the time.

Whichever qualitative method you choose, FuelTarget™ or Periodization Plates™, remember that the main goals are to con-trol your blood sugar, improve satiety, and use the concept of thermogenesis to aid in your weight goals.

STEP 3: USE QUANTITATIVE METHODS BUT WISELY

Quantitative Weight-Loss Approaches

This approach is for the athlete who likes numbers and tracking quantitative data and trends. For athletes of the opposite nature, you may want to stop here and spend your time in the instinctual or qualitative sections because they may be more successful for you. Remember, however, that you can certainly combine a few strategies from each to best suit your style and meet your needs.

Overall, losing weight and body fat is really not that difficult when you see it described on paper. However, for most athletes, weight loss is more complex than balancing the number of calories that go in the body with the number of calories that leave the body. If it were not complex, athletes would never encounter failure. The hard truth is that food is a crutch for many athletes. Stress, emotions, and boredom can all influence what, when, why, and how much you eat. And you know as well as I do that stress levels can rise quickly, boredom can set in without blinking an eye, and emotions, well, they can take you on a roller coaster ride from minute to minute throughout the day.

I don't know if it is realistic to ask you to master your mind, but if you can get a good handle on your thought processes and emotions, you can do a better job at managing your body. Don't strive for perfection. Strive for life balance.

You may well have heard the saying "a calorie is a calorie." Is it true? Well, according to the energy balance equation, the answer is yes. However, looking more deeply into the metabolic rate of foods, you learn that certain macronutrients have a different thermic effect. Let me help you understand this concept and how it can work to your benefit. When you eat a food, your body must metabolize it to be able to use it. The process of metabolism generates heat (the next time you eat a meal, notice whether you feel warmer toward the end of the meal). The more heat you produce, the more calories your body loses.

As described earlier, each of the macronutrients has a different thermic effect. Carbohydrates and protein contain 4 calories per gram and fat contains 9 calories per gram, but because each exhibits a different thermic effect on the body, "all calories are equal" simply cannot be a true statement when you are looking at when the food is consumed and how it is metabolized. Remember, simple means sustainable. Don't spend too much time trying to digest this concept fully (pun intended!). The important take-home message is that macronutrients produce different thermic effects when metabolized, and you can use that to your advantage when trying to manipulate your body weight.

A paradigm shift to eating supports a more balanced macronutrient distribution, which, for many athletes, means cutting down on the bland color carbohydrates and increasing the lean meats and meat alternatives. Let me now engage you in the quantitative side of weight loss. But remember, this is the last step in losing weight, and for good reason. If you choose to use this method, be sure that you are ready for it and have spent some time in the first two steps. This helps ensure that you are not overwhelmed by the numbers and that you can actually use some of the information from quantitative assessment and analysis.

Energy Balance Equation

The first step in this weight-loss option is to manipulate what I call your Personal Energy Balance Equation (PEBE). The energy balance equation has two components: calories-in (consumption) and calories-out (expenditure), as shown in Figure 4.1. The calories-in side is made up of foodstuffs that you consume. More specifically, these include the following:

- Carbohydrate
- Protein
- Fat
- Alcohol

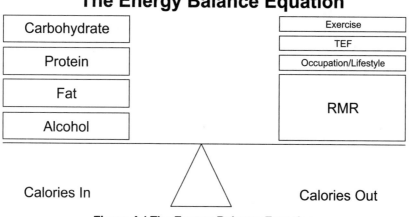

The Energy Balance Equation

Carbohydrate		Exercise
Protein		TEF
Fat		Occupation/Lifestyle
Alcohol		RMR

Calories In   Calories Out

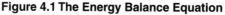

Figure 4.1 The Energy Balance Equation

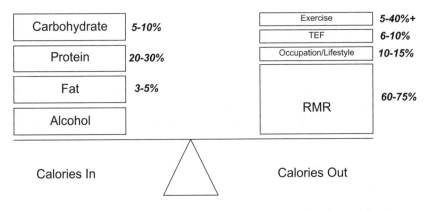

Figure 4.2 Energy balance equation, the thermatic effect of food and energy and energy expenditure

This side of the equation appears to be simple to understand because it is only affected by the amount and types of food you eat or beverages you drink. However, each macronutrient (alcohol is not considered a macronutrient; therefore I do not address it) has a different thermic effect in the body (see Figure 4.2).

The calories-out side of the energy balance equation is much more complicated because biology has more of an impact on each component. You can look at a nutrition facts label on a food product and know with somewhat close accuracy how many calories you would be consuming. Unfortunately, there is more guess work when it comes to the right side of your PEBE. The factors that comprise this side of the energy balance equation include the following:

- Thermic effect of food (TEF)
- Occupational and lifestyle expenditure
- Exercise expenditure
- Resting metabolic rate (RMR)

Similar to the calories-in side, each of the four components on the calories-out side has a different contribution to the total number of calories that you burn or expend.

Thermic Effect of Food

Although some textbooks state that TEF can be approximately 10% of your total energy expenditure, it can vary greatly, depending on both the quantity and quality of food that you eat. TEF is certainly not the magic bullet of weight loss, but you can use TEF as one of the tools needed to manipulate your weight successfully. TEF actually has its own subsets, which are important for you to understand:

- ○ Obligatory thermogenesis: the number of calories that your body burns as it digests and absorbs the food that you eat.
- ○ Facultative thermogenesis: occurs when your nervous system gets activated from eating and increases your metabolism.

Occupational/Lifestyle Expenditure

Occupational/lifestyle expenditure can make up approximately 10–15% of the total calories that you burn each day. You can have a significant impact on the amount of weight or body fat that you lose by taking advantage of this. What I mean is that regardless of what type of occupation you have or what you do during the day, you have the ability to take more steps, park farther away from the front door, make more trips to the water fountain, or take the stairs. You can do all this without having to plan as you do with your training. The calories you can burn—in your normal day, outside of training—can almost be referred to as "free calories" because you don't have to change clothes, sweat, or follow a structured training program to burn them. The more calories you burn in your daily non-training activities, the more a caloric deficit you can create.

Certainly, society in general does not make this easy and does not encourage or reward this type of behavior. Without stepping on my soapbox and preaching to the choir, it is important to understand that although this component may seem easy and may provide you with "free" calorie-burning opportunities, it does require a strong effort to accomplish. Imagine that you work on the fourth floor of an office building and you arrive to work at the same time as your colleagues. You enter the lobby and your co-workers gravitate toward the elevator. You know that you want to take the stairs to increase your daily calorie expenditure. Do you choose the elevator and follow the norm, or do you choose the stairs and step outside the norm? Regardless of which you choose, it is a tough decision the first few times you make it. However, rest assured that choosing the method that best assists you with your weight-loss goals does not label you as an outcast. In fact, you may find that, over time, more of your co-workers join you!

Another very simple method of attempting to increase the number of calories that you burn throughout the day through occupational and/or lifestyle activity is the use of a step-counter, or pedometer. These devices track the amount of steps that you take during the day, are very cost-effective, and are extremely easy to use. In general, it can be assumed that most people take between 2,000–2,500 steps per mile walked. Using the general calculation that 100 calories are burned for each mile walked, it is possible to burn in excess of 500 calories per day simply by taking a very unstructured and very simplistic approach to weight loss. If you work in an office where meetings are more frequent than pit stops to the bathroom, you are very challenged to even acquire 5,000 steps. But remember, weight loss doesn't come easy. Take the bull by the horns, be accountable for your actions, and make it happen. You have the choice to use this piece of the energy balance equation to your benefit or not.

Exercise Expenditure

Exercise expenditure is the most variable component of the calories-out side that over which you have control. What I mean is that you can burn as few as 5% or as many as 40% of your total calories through exercise, depending on the frequency, intensity, time, and type of exercise that you perform. If you have a somewhat structured training program, this will be easy. Simply follow your program. Can you introduce more exercise to get a higher calorie burn? Sure, but just be careful when you do so that you do not risk overtraining or injury. Many weight-class athletes introduce more exercise frequently and with great success.

Resting Metabolic Rate

Resting metabolic rate (RMR) is the number of calories that your body burns at rest to perform basic functions such as proper heart and brain functioning. Don't get resting confused with basal metabolic rate (often referred to as BMR or basal energy expenditure BEE). RMR is typically 5–10% higher than BMR because it involves a rested state, not a basal state. Accurately measuring BMR requires a hospital setting where movement before testing is minimal. The benefit of RMR is that it can comprise approximately 60–75% of the number of calories that you burn each day. RMR is certainly the greatest energy expenditure component on the calories-out side of the energy balance equation because it represents up to three-quarters of the total calories burned by the body.

To use RMR accurately in your energy balance equation, it should be measured. Remember, this is the quantitative approach to weight loss, and you want to be as exact as possible. You need to find a health-care facility, such as a hospital, or a fitness center or healthcare provider, such as a Registered Dietitian or Exercise Physiologist to have your RMR measured.

Even more important is the pre-RMR protocol, which, when not followed, can produce significant errors. I have performed hundreds of RMR tests and have consistently found that athletes who do not follow the protocol typically have higher RMRs. This small "error" can mean the difference between weight-loss success or failure. In fact, research has proven that the calorie difference can range from 200 to 1,000 calories when a proper protocol is not followed.

You should also know that, although a facility or provider offers RMR measurements, protocols can differ. The key to measuring any biological function (cholesterol, blood pressure, resting heart rate, etc.) is accuracy and consistency. If you want to have your RMR measured, I highly recommend the following protocol:

1. Measure the RMR first thing in the morning. Minimize movement to the facility where you have it measured.
2. Do not eat anything with calories or caffeine for at least 12 hours before the measurement.
3. Do not exercise (strength or aerobic) for at least 12 hours before the measurement.
4. Do not have your RMR measured if you are getting sick, are sick, or are taking acute medications for an illness.
5. Do not use nicotine for at least 4 hours before the measurement.
6. Relax in a comfortable position for 15–20 minutes before the measurement begins.

Once you have met this protocol, be sure that you follow these guidelines during your measurement:

1. Sit or lie in a comfortable chair or on a mat in a relaxed environment, with dim lights and a thermoneutral environment (not too warm, not too cold).
2. Breathe normally and do not manipulate your breathing patterns.
3. Do not fall asleep.
4. Try not to cough, sneeze, or move. Remain as still as possible.

Depending on the machine that is used to measure your RMR and the facility's protocol, you can expect the test to take from 5–30 minutes not including the rest time beforehand.

If you know your measured RMR, you can build a more exact calorie budget that provides you with enough energy to train and lose weight and body fat. The energy balance equation is a good place to begin to learn about the different factors that affect your weight-loss rate and success. However, because of the large psychological component to weight loss, focusing on calories-in versus calories-out is not the only piece of the weight-loss puzzle. It is merely one piece of the puzzle.

Once you are ready and want to use this quantitative approach to weight loss, you can have your RMR measured. I have had many athletes ask me if it is okay to use one of those fancy metabolic calculators or equations to estimate their RMR. My answer is simple. If you are going to use this more exact approach to weight loss, you cannot rely on an estimate that can have an error range of 200–1,000 calories. If you have an analytical personality, you thrive on numbers. Go have your RMR measured, and leave no stone unturned. As I mentioned earlier, it is crucial to control as many external factors as possible before having your RMR measured. Even the measurement that you obtain is not 100% accurate. But think about it, nothing is! Body composition? No! It doesn't matter which method you use: dual energy x-ray absorptiometry (DEXA), hydrostatic weighing, air displacement, or skinfold calipers. There is still some degree of error. Cholesterol? No? Have you ever had your blood drawn and submitted to two different labs? If you haven't, you would be shocked to find out that the values would likely not be the same. In fact, they could be off enough to qualify you as high at one lab and normal at the other. The fact is that you cannot control biology entirely. It changes every millisecond. However, what you can do is control some of the external factors that affect it. Estimating your RMR is useless because it is affected by so many different factors that equations don't account for. Specifically, RMR is influenced by these factors:

- Mass: the more you weigh, the higher your RMR. An easy way to think about this is using the analogy of a large, gas-guzzling SUV versus a smaller, more gas-economical car. The SUV requires and takes more gas to move than does the smaller car. It is the same thing with your body. When you weigh more, you need more calories to survive. When you weigh less, you don't need as many calories.

- Body composition: the more muscle you have, the higher your RMR.
- Gender: males usually have higher RMRs because they have more lean muscle mass.
- Genetics: it is believed that RMR can be affected by as much as 30% depending on your genetics.
- Medications: some drugs increase RMR, but others decrease it.
- Hormones: stress hormones, in particular, typically increase your RMR.

Measuring RMR

Because the number one factor that influences your RMR is your body mass, a loss of body weight causes a decrease in your RMR and vice versa. When you lose weight, your RMR also decreases. This explains the infamous "yo-yo" dieting phenomenon that happens with athletes trying to lose weight: they decrease the number of calories that they eat, which results in weight loss. But their RMR decreases at the same time because they are now at a lower body weight. Normally, this is not a cause for concern—except when the athletes look in the mirror, like what they see from the weight they have lost, and decide to celebrate by eating a couple of cookies, going out for a big dinner celebration with friends, or missing a few training sessions. Those athletes are now increasing the calories-in side of their PEBE, and guess what? Their new, lower RMR has a hard time catching back up to support this new increased calorie level. Because RMR cannot catch up at the same rate as the calories are going in or not being burned, they begin to gain weight again.

Having your RMR measured on a consistent basis is the most important thing you can do when you are trying to lose weight. I cannot stress enough how important it is to get your new RMR measured whenever you lose about 10% of your total body weight or when you reach a weight-loss plateau.

The only accurate method to have your RMR measured is to visit a performance center or health professional that has an indirect calorimeter, commonly called a metabolic cart. Check your local physician's office, a registered dietitian, or a health club to see if they have the capability of measuring your RMR. Remember, you want to have your RMR measured with a device that you breathe into, not estimated using an equation based on your gender, age, height, and weight.

After you find a qualified health professional to measure your RMR, here is what you can expect from the measurement process itself. A machine measures the volume of oxygen (resting VO_2) that you breathe in and out. The test itself is very noninvasive because you simply have to breathe. You sit quietly and comfortably with a mouthpiece in your mouth or under what is called a ventilated hood that collects the oxygen and, possibly, carbon dioxide (depending on the machine) that you inspire and expire and then analyzes it. It can take from 5–30 minutes; after it is done, you know how many calories your body needs in a 24-hour period just to maintain itself at its current weight.

After having this piece of information, the next step is to meet with a registered dietitian (RD) who specializes in sports nutrition. Search for a qualified Sport Dietitian at www.scandpg .org. Be sure to look for the initials CSSD after an RD's name. Being a Board Certified Specialist in Sports Dietetics (CSSD) ensures that this person has experience working with athletes. He or she will be able to assist you with feeding appropriately based on the demands of your sport relative to your weight-loss goals.

The Sport Dietitian may ask you to log the food and beverages that you consume in order to calculate numbers based on your RMR measurement. As you read in the beginning of this chapter, I am not the biggest fan of calorie counting, but it can be useful in the early stages of using the quantitative approach. In fact, keeping a food log can improve your awareness of food, along with keeping you more accountable. Just be sure to maintain a balance without becoming a slave to the numbers each and every day of your life. Use food logging in the beginning once you have a good handle on the instinctual and qualitative steps to weight loss. At the same time, it is useful to monitor your exercise expenditure through a heart rate monitor or portable energy expenditure device. Understanding both sides of the energy balance equation is important when using the quantitative approach.

A significant change in RMR from one measurement to the next is 100–200 calories—as long as you have it measured by the same device, the same person, at the same time of day, same time of the month, and under the same fasting conditions. Readjust your PEBE only if your RMR is different by at least 100 calories or more or if you have been at a weight plateau for more than seven days. If your PEBE is not readjusted with each RMR measurement, it is difficult for you to remain successful at attaining your weight-related goals. For example, one 12-week weight-loss study showed that at week 4, participants had lost 8 pounds and RMR had decreased by 89 calories. If the participants did not readjust the number of calories they ate and expended, they would not continue to lose weight. In fact, the researchers in this study readjusted the energy balance equation at certain intervals, and, at week 12, the average weight loss was 18 pounds, with a decrease in RMR of 125 calories. This shows that a very small decrease in RMR can make a big difference in adjusting your PEBE for continuing to lose weight.

Case Study for Weight Loss

Let's look at an example so that you have an idea of how it all fits together.

Julie is a master swimmer who focuses on long course competitions and wants to eventually try open water racing. She is 5'4" and weighs 150 pounds; she wants to lose 20 pounds, and she has just started her 16-week pre-season.

Julie visited a registered dietitian (RD) and had her RMR measured. Her RMR was 1,300 calories per day. She then met with the RD to fill in the remaining components of her PEBE, working on the calories-out side first.

In terms of occupational and lifestyle expenditure, Julie works in an office on a computer, eight hours per day, five days per week, so it was determined that the number of calories that she burned during work were minimal. For a relatively sedentary occupation, the number of calories burned is around 600 per day.

For her exercise expenditure, Julie trains six days per week. She swims eight hours per week and lifts weights for two hours per week. Based on these amounts of planned exercise, she burns approximately:

- Swimming: 3,860 calories per week
- Strength training: 450 calories per week

Julie's total calories burned through exercise are 4,310 per week or 615 calories per day. There are many books and Web sites that can provide you with the tools to calculate how many calories you burn when you exercise, and I recommend consulting these to figure out your specific energy expenditure because it is dependent upon body weight, duration, and intensity of exercise.

After determining that Julie burns 2,515 calories per day (1,300 from her RMR, 600 from her occupation, 615 from her exercise), it was time to determine how many calories she should eat per day.

By setting the number of calories that she eats per day at between 1,600–1,800, Julie will be in a negative energy balance, which should begin her weight loss. Although many athletes have heard that 3,500 calories equals 1 pound of weight, this does not always hold true, as described earlier. Thus, creating a calorie deficit of 500 per day to equal a 3,500-calorie deficit in 1 week will not be adhered to because of the inaccuracy. Rather, providing Julie with enough of the proper calories to keep her full and to satisfy her hunger and training needs based on her training cycle is the main goal in the beginning phases.

Some things to keep in mind about this example:

1. Because Julie is just beginning her pre-season, which includes lower volume and intensity, she does not need to eat as many

calories. Once her training volume begins to increase throughout this cycle, she can begin to even out the deficit between the calories that she eats and the calories that she burns.

2. Because of the lower training load, Julie could eat as few as 1,300 calories per day if she really wanted to because this is was her measured RMR and the calories needed to sustain life processes. I often ask athletes with whom I work how aggressive they want to be and how motivated they are to lose the weight. If both answers are positive, I reduce their daily calorie intake to around 200–300 calories above their measured RMR to begin with and then closely monitor their training status, sleep patterns, and immune system. However, it is important to never eat fewer calories than your RMR for too long (more than a couple of days) because it sends your body into starvation response mode, and you likely store more fat and won't lose weight, even though you are eating less. It is your body's way of protecting itself.

Now that Julie has a better idea of how many calories she should eat, based on her individual RMR, she can begin to apply this information as she makes food choices. Julie has a couple of options:

- The first is to use a computer-based food-logging program where she can log all of her food and beverage intake. This is a nice option because it provides somewhat accurate data; however, it is not a good fit for some athletes. Determine whether using a computer fits your lifestyle and personality and whether you would take the time to use it to log your calorie intake. If you do not devote the time each day to log your food, it is not worth doing.
- What I usually recommend is that athletes read nutrition labels on the foods they eat and that they write down the calorie content per serving that they eat for about 7–10 days. This exercise teaches them the calorie content of common foods and allows them to keep track of their calorie levels. I

also recommend doing this exercise every 2–4 weeks as a refresher and to make sure that they still have a good grasp of the calories that they are eating.

Julie can log her exercise via a computer software program, or she can use the pencil-and-paper method.

- When you use the pencil-and-paper method, the numbers are not as accurate, so I recommend at least using an online resource or calorie-counting book that provides calories burned for different exercises.

Julie can easily keep track of her occupational activity calories burned by wearing a step-counter. A step-counter, worn throughout the day, provides her with the number of steps that she takes so that she can figure out the number of calories that her body burns during nonpurposeful activity.

Eight weeks later, Julie has lost 10 pounds. She has her RMR measured again to discover that it is 1,200 calories. This is completely normal; the number one predictor of RMR is body mass.

With her new RMR, she visits the RD again to readjust her PEBE so that she does not get stuck on a weight plateau or start gaining weight.

The quantitative step is certainly more number crunching, but it provides you a different perspective on weight loss from a number-driven model. As I mentioned earlier in this chapter, this step is the last in the process, for good reason. Athletes who begin with the calorie-counting method often do not see long-term success. Ignoring the instinctual and qualitative aspects associated with food leads to much frustration in the future.

Weight-Loss Timing

Because of the many sport classifications that exist, ranging from endurance to strength to team to weight-classified, there is not an ideal time of the training year to pursue weight loss. Athletes in certain sports know when the time is right. What I can say as a general recommendation is that unless you compete in a weight-classified sport such as wrestling, boxing, or tae kwon do, there really isn't an "ideal" time to pursue weight loss.

There are many factors associated with implementing a successful weight-loss plan, as you have learned throughout this chapter. Once the instinctual and emotional connections with food are engaged and being actively pursued, it is much easier to stare the weight-loss monster in the eyes because you will have much more self-confidence and trust in yourself.

Endurance athletes may seek weight loss during their pre-season, whereas athletes performing team and strength sports may attempt it during their off-season. The training cycle and physical goals for each specific cycle must be taken into consideration before engaging in weight loss. The worst thing for any athlete to have happen is a decrement in performance, immune system health, or sleep quality, all of which have a negative impact on performance and recovery.

My primary recommendation to you as you embark on the weight-loss journey is to begin at Step 1 and do not shortchange yourself by neglecting the importance of it. This, along with understanding the qualities of food and their impact on your appetite, as described in Step 2, is absolutely necessary for ensuring long-term success in any of your weight-loss goals throughout your sport career.

Weight Gain

Certainly weight gain is not as popular for athletes as weight loss. However, as strange as it may sound, some athletes have a very tough time either maintaining or gaining weight. These athletes are typically the weight lifters or wrestlers, who are trying to move up a weight class or be at the highest weight in their class; the football players, who are trying to get bigger for better performance; or, on the other end of the continuum, the female endurance athlete who has been amenorrheic and needs to increase the number of calories that she eats in order for her body to regain menses. The common theme is that weight gain is needed to improve performance and/or health, and these athletes may have just as difficult a time doing this as do the athletes who are trying to lose weight.

These athletes often have a high RMR, which can be a product of the genetic deck of cards that they were dealt, their body type/structure, their sport of choice, or a combination of some or all. Although the reason why the body cannot seem to maintain or gain weight is intriguing and sometimes mysterious, even more important is the "how" behind achieving this goal.

It may seem easy to tell athletes simply to eat more calories in a day, but what is often overlooked is how many calories their body is expending during training and daily activities. A great example of this was an elite male weight lifter I knew who was desperately trying to gain weight. Because he had so much trouble with this, he drove as close as even a few hundred feet to appointments and training sessions to avoid burning too many calories walking. He also took the elevator instead of the stairs for this same reason.

FuelStory #3

An example at the opposite end of the continuum is that of a female marathoner who was having astounding results and wanted to continue this trend. However, she was amenorrheic and had low bone-mineral density. These conditions are extremely unhealthy, but, because she was performing well, she did not realize that there was an issue that was negatively affecting her health. The difficultly was proving to this athlete that this was a problem and that if it was not addressed, she might not be able to compete in the future. An increase in calories was needed, but, because her performance level was high, she did not accept the higher-calorie prescription, nor did she follow it.

Another great example that is quite common involved a competitive male swimmer who, for the life of him, lost weight yet ate six times per day—and not small portions! Some swimmers train twice a day and spend upward of 4–6 hours in the pool daily, not including their dry-land and strength-training programs. His inability to maintain his weight had a negative impact on his performance. He knew that he needed to put on weight to improve his performance, but he could not seem to do it no matter how much he ate. Simply telling him to eat more food did not work.

Weight-gain goals share a striking resemblance to those of weight loss. Changing habits and forming new behaviors are the focal areas. Take the example of the female marathoner. Weight gain was needed for health reasons, but she was either not cognizant that this was a concern or she was not ready to make a change because her performance was high. Regardless of the reason, the bottom line was that she might not be able to continue competing at this level of performance for long because her health could be compromised. I have seen many athletes in the same situation; what usually happens is that an extended illness or injury provides the "wake-up" call. Unfortunately, it is often too late. Athletes may miss their season or quality training time, which affects performance. The most important intervention with such athletes is for close friends or family members to provide positive support and to express their concern for the athlete's health. This begins the process, and although this is certainly not going to fix the problem, it allows the athletes to acknowledge that their health is being compromised. Then they can progress through the series of stages in the Stages of Change Model. These athletes, by far, are the most challenging to work with when it comes to weight gain. I encourage them to take baby steps along the way because those are typically more successful and less overwhelming.

The example of the male competitive swimmer requires a completely different approach. It is important that you understand the intervention differences: each requires a different set of skills when managing weight gain. This athlete has no health concerns. Rather, weight gain is needed to improve his performance, and he knows it. He is ready to take the steps, but with less success than he had hoped. This is as simple as restructuring the quality of the calories that he is eating. For this athlete and any other seeking weight gain, it is important to create a daily positive energy balance. That is, eating more calories than the body is expending. It does sound easy, I'll give it that, but the problem I encounter the most is that athletes in this scenario eat fairly "clean" (nutrient-dense, low-refined sugars, higher fiber). Even though I am a big proponent of eating "clean," it can cause an athlete to undereat because of a higher nutrient density and fiber intake. Eating a diet that is higher in fiber is extremely beneficial for health, but, because of the increased roughage in the diet, the athletes stay feeling fuller longer, which means that even if they are eating six times per day, they are not eating enough calories. By adding a higher calorie beverage (what I call a "supersmoothie") in the daily eating regimen, it is possible to increase their weight. I normally recommend a liquid beverage that contains around 1,000 calories. The liquid source is important because it does not provide the bulk of solid food; therefore, the athletes can consume it without much problem. They should drink it throughout the day, not in one sitting. The important thing is that they be consistent in drinking it every day until their reach their weight goal.

Amount of Weight Loss

There is really no ideal weight loss per week; it is highly dependent upon the athlete. Losing between 0.5–1.0 pounds per week minimizes losses of muscle glycogen and lean muscle mass, compromised cardiac function, altered ability to maintain body temperature, and muscle cramping as a result of electrolyte imbalances. However, some athletes have good success with losing between 1.0–4.0 pounds per week.

Because frequent changes in scale weight (5 pounds or less) typically reflect changes in fluid balance or glycogen stores, focus more on changes in your body composition and girth measurements rather than on your total body weight. The best method to use is via skin calipers with tracking absolute millimeters pinched at each site rather than percentage of body fat. The latter simply does not track changes in different parts of your body as well. Different equations are used to calculate percentage of body fat, and you cannot have an accurate representation of where your body is storing, gaining, or losing most of its fat. There is about 2–4% inaccuracy when reporting body fat percentage based on equations. Girth measurements, combined with absolute millimeters taken via skinfold calipers, are the easiest way to track trends, and both measurements can be done very easily every 4–6 weeks.

SUMMARY

Food is fuel. However, eating isn't as easy as pulling into the gas station and filling up your car with gas. Food is around you frequently throughout the day, and it provides great temptation. This makes it more difficult to manage, hence the high incidences of emotional eating patterns. I have helped hundreds of athletes lose weight and a good handful of them gain weight—on purpose, don't worry! You can and will be successful if you adopt the principles presented in this chapter.

Remember, to change your behavior, you must first be in the right stage of change, which provides you with the proper motivation for changing behaviors and habits. Control your mind, and you control your body. Then tackle the instinctual component of weight management, and you will be on the road to improving your self-confidence and trust, both of which are necessary components in the weight-loss or weight-gain journey.

5

Nutrition Supplementation

Should I take it? Do I need it? Is it safe? Does it work? How much does it cost? These are the most common questions I hear from athletes about nutritional supplements. I address most of these questions in this chapter and help you determine whether you should add a nutritional supplement to your daily eating program.

This chapter provides you with information regarding some of the more popular nutrition supplements used by athletes as well as information about common ingredients found in nutrition supplements. Ingredients education is often overlooked by athletes, but if you have a better understanding of what types of ingredients are being added to your favorite supplements, you will have a better understanding about how they work in your body and you can decide which ones are right for you and your specific needs. But first, let's take a look at nutritional supplements in general.

THE NUTRITION SUPPLEMENTS MARKET

Nutrition supplements are probably one of the most popular training aids among athletes. I am confident in stating that every athlete takes some type of supplement—ranging from a simple multi-vitamin to a complex assortment of pills, powders, and potions. The reason is simple: supplements encompass a wider range of products than most athletes think. I discuss this in more detail later in the chapter, but remember that a supplement is something that is added to a diet that is comprised of food and drink.

Open up an athlete's pantry and I can almost guarantee that you'll find a bottle of multi-vitamins, a tub of a sports drink or recovery beverage, a few boxes of energy bars, and possibly even some "mystery" supplements that promise unrealistic claims. Supplements are real. You use them, and I am not going to try to change your mind because some do truly have a role in sport. However, it is your responsibility to choose supplements that are safe and legal. It helps if they actually work, but if you experience a placebo effect from a safe and legal supplement, who am I to tell you that you cannot use it? You may be wasting your money, but if it is not compromising your health, performance, or eligibility to play your sport, it could indeed be an ergogenic aid.

If you can tell, I am quite liberal and open about supplements. I have worked with far too many athletes to be naïve about this topic. Supplements are part of sport. It is my duty to help you navigate the good ones from the bad ones. Take any athlete as an example, and you'll find justification for taking a multi-vitamin during certain training cycles when training load is high. There are additional supplements that can be extremely beneficial to even the most elite athletes, as long as they are taken in the right doses at the right time and for the right reasons. I explain this in more detail later in the chapter. First, let me discuss supplement industry regulation, or lack thereof in some instances, to give you a better idea of the problem that exists surrounding supplements.

SUPPLEMENT REGULATION

I understand that this information may not be on the top of your "want to learn" list, but I believe that it is relevant in order for you to have the foundation knowledge of the supplement market as a whole.

The Dietary Supplements Health and Education Act (DSHEA) of 1994 states that nutritional supplements that do not claim to diagnose, prevent, or cure disease are not subject to regulation by the Food and Drug Administration (FDA). Unfortunately many supplement manufacturers have concluded that DSHEA guidelines mean that there is no need for them to prove claimed benefits, to show safety with acute or chronic administration, to commit to accepted quality assurance practices, or to follow the stringent labeling regulations followed for food products.

As a result, dietary ingredients used in dietary supplements are no longer subject to the pre-market safety evaluations required of other new food ingredients or for new uses of old food ingredients. The intent of DSHEA was to meet the concerns of manufacturers and consumers to help ensure that safe and well-labeled products were available to individuals who wanted to use them.

The purposes of DSHEA included the following:

1. Define dietary supplements and dietary ingredients.
   - Through the DSHEA, Congress expanded the meaning of the term "dietary supplements" beyond essential nutrients to include such substances as ginseng, garlic, fish oils, psyllium, enzymes, glandulars, and mixtures of these.
   - The DSHEA defined "dietary supplement" as a product (other than tobacco) that is intended to supplement the diet that bears or contains one or more of the following dietary ingredients: a vitamin, a mineral, an herb or other botanical, an amino acid, a dietary substance for use by humans to supplement the diet by increasing the total daily intake, concentrate, metabolite, constituent, extract, or combinations of these ingredients.
   - Dietary supplements are intended for ingestion in pill, capsule, tablet, or liquid form; are not represented for use as a conventional food or as the sole item of a meal or diet; must be labeled as a "dietary supplement"; and include products such as an approved new drug, certified

antibiotic, or licensed biologic that was marketed as a dietary supplement or food before approval, certification, or license.

2. Establish a new framework for assuring safety.
   - Under DSHEA, a dietary supplement is contaminated if one or more of its ingredients presents "a significant or unreasonable risk of illness or injury" when used as directed on the label, or under normal conditions of use. It is a manufacturer's responsibility to ensure that its products are safe and properly labeled prior to marketing.

3. Outline guidelines for literature are displayed where supplements are sold.
   - The DSHEA provides that retail outlets may make available third-party materials to help inform consumers about any health-related benefits of dietary supplements. These materials can include articles, book chapters, or scientific abstracts. These provisions state that the information must not be false or misleading, cannot promote a specific supplement brand, must be displayed with other similar materials to present a balanced view, and must be displayed separately from supplements.

4. Provide for use of claims and nutritional support statements.
   - The DSHEA provides for the use of various types of statements on the label of dietary supplements, although claims may not be made about the use of a dietary supplement to diagnose, prevent, mitigate, treat, or cure a specific disease. Under DSHEA, firms can make statements about classical nutrient deficiency diseases as long as these statements disclose the prevalence of the disease in the United States. In addition, manufacturers may describe the supplement's effects on "structure or function" of the body or the "well-being" achieved by using the dietary ingredient. To use these claims, manufacturers must have substantiation that the statements are truthful and not misleading, and the

product label must bear the statement: "This statement has not been evaluated by the Food and Drug Administration. This product is not intended to diagnose, treat, cure, or prevent any disease." Unlike health claims, nutritional support statements need not be approved by the FDA before manufacturers market products bearing the statements.

5. Require ingredient and nutrition labeling; grant the FDA the authority to establish good manufacturing practice (GMP) regulations.

    ○ Like other foods, dietary supplement products must have ingredient labels. This information must include the name and quantity of each dietary ingredient and identify the product as a "dietary supplement." Labeling of products containing herbal and botanical ingredients must state the part of the plant from which the ingredient is derived. If a supplement is covered by specifications in an official compendium and is represented as conforming, it is misbranded if it does not conform to those specifications. Official compendia include the U.S. Pharmacopeia, the Homeopathic Pharmacopeia of the United States, or the National Formulary. If not covered by a compendium, a dietary supplement must be the product identified on the label and have the strength that it is represented as having.

    ○ Labels also must provide nutrition labeling. This labeling must first list dietary ingredients present in "significant amounts" for which the FDA has established daily consumption recommendations, followed by dietary ingredients with no daily intake recommendations. Dietary ingredients that are not present in significant amounts need not be listed. The nutrition labeling must include the quantity per serving for each dietary ingredient (or proprietary blend) and may include the source of a dietary ingredient. If an ingredient is listed in the nutrition labeling, it does not need to appear in the statement of ingredients. Nutrition information must precede ingredient statements on the product label.

○ DSHEA grants the FDA the authority to establish GMP regulations governing the preparation, packing, and holding of dietary supplements under conditions that ensure their safety. These regulations are to be modeled after current good manufacturing practice regulations in effect for the rest of the food industry. The FDA intends to work with the supplement industry and other interested persons to develop GMPs and, in doing so, seeks public comment as to their scope.

The nutritional supplement industry represents a multibillion dollar per year growth industry. Interestingly, the industry is moving toward compiling more scientific data and validation of products and claims for formulation and marketing purposes. Because of this, companies continue to outsource their production to contract manufacturers who already have good quality control procedures and laboratories in place. What this means for athletes is a better chance of having noncontaminated supplement products, although, as the following makes clear, the risk of supplement contamination is always present and should always be taken seriously regardless of which supplement is considered.

SUPPLEMENT CONTAMINATION

Athletes from around the world are turning to nutritional supplements as a way to get bigger, faster, and stronger and to get any possible edge over their competition. However, what athletes do not know—or are finding out the hard way—is that many of the supplements on the shelves do not contain the advertised amounts of substances in them or, even worse, have additional substances in them that are not listed on the label. This can be of particular concern if you have health issues such that a certain herbal product or manufactured supplement could interfere with medications that you may be taking.

Quality assurance for dietary supplements continues to be a concern. Some companies follow GMPs, but others do not. It is difficult to know what products contain, especially when you consider that contamination of a supplement can occur at so many levels in the supply and manufacturing process. If you try to reduce your risk by avoiding all products of companies that produce and sell prohormones, such as nandrolone and testosterone derivatives that result in positive drug tests, this may still not be enough protection.

Since the release of the Schanzer report, commissioned by the International Olympic Committee in 1999, which stated that 18% of all dietary supplements may lead to a positive doping offense, there has been increasing commercial awareness of the adverse publicity that companies face if they are connected with contaminated products. As discussed in the following, these products are not limited to supplements that only benefit strength and power athletes. You may be surprised to see some of the common supplements that you take may be at risk for supplement contamination.

The problem is clearly widespread, as indicated by an investigation conducted by the International Olympic Committee laboratory in Cologne, Germany. During 2000 and 2001, 634 supplements from 13 different countries were purchased and tested. Of these, 94 supplements (14.8% of the total) contained prohibited substances. It was indicated that in another 10% steroids may have been present, but the analysis was not conclusive. These results point to a risk of contamination with prohibited substances of one in four!

Products that tested positive were purchased in the Netherlands (26%), Austria (23%), the United States (19%), the United Kingdom (19%), Italy (14%), Spain (14%), and Germany (12%), among others. Contamination levels of products tended to be small and highly variable among and within batches, making it difficult to identify the source of the contaminated supplement. Even though the prohibited substances that were found have not been officially published, they included the following types and/or categories:

- Branched-chain amino acids (popular among endurance athletes)
- Glutamine (popular among endurance athletes)
- Zinc (popular among endurance athletes)
- Chrysin
- Tribulus terrestris
- Vitamins (popular among endurance athletes)
- Minerals (popular among endurance athletes)
- Antioxidants
- Creatine
- Ribose
- Conjugated linoleic acid
- Carnitine
- Guarana
- Pyruvate
- Beta-hydroxy-beta-methylbutyrate (HMB)
- Protein powders (popular among endurance athletes)
- Herbal extracts

There are several industry-driven GMP programs in place, although many experts continue to be concerned about sources of raw materials and guarantees for each batch of product. One industry program is overseen by the National Nutritional Foods Association (NNFA), which has certified dozens of companies and has a strategic alliance with NSF International (www.nsf.org). Membership in NNFA requires compliance with its GMPs, and its Web site (www.nnfa.org) lists companies that are members. NSF International has an athlete-certification program and can test specific products for interested athletes. Other resources include consumerlab.com, which has independently tested dietary supplements and has an Athletic Banned Substances Screened Products

Program; the FDA, which has also presented an outline of a GMP program on its Web site at www.cfsan.fda.gov; and Informed Choice (www.informed-choice.org).

I am not suggesting that you avoid all nutritional supplements. However, it is important to exercise caution when choosing supplements because any product can be contaminated; industry standards are not in place to prevent this. Any product has the risk of being contaminated, even a simple multi-vitamin.

WHAT TO LOOK FOR AND WHAT TO AVOID

You are constantly faced with new supplements that claim to improve aerobic capacity, buffer lactic acid, decrease muscle soreness, increase strength and power, improve recovery, improve lean muscle mass, and improve immune function. This list goes on and on, but which ones really work is the question to ask before taking any one of them. There are a few ergogenic (performance-enhancing) aids that have withstood the rigors of time and scientific testing for which the claims have been substantiated, but the majority of ergogenic aids have no proven research to support their claims. Before I discuss popular supplements used by athletes, I want to provide you with a 12-step checklist to help you decide whether a product is truly worth buying. If you answer yes to any of these questions, you should be skeptical of such supplements and investigate them further before buying them.

1. Does the product promise quick improvement in health or physical performance?
2. Does it contain some secret ingredient or formula?
3. Is it advertised mainly with anecdotes, case histories, or testimonials?
4. Are currently popular personalities or star athletes featured in its advertisements?
5. Does it take a simple truth about a nutrient and exaggerate that truth in terms of health or physical performance?

196 Nutrition Periodization for Endurance Athletes

6. Does it question the integrity of the scientific or medical establishment?
7. Is it advertised in a health or sports magazine by publishers who also sell nutritional aids?
8. Does the person who recommends it also sell the product?
9. Does it use the results of a single study or outdated and poorly controlled research to support its claims?
10. Is it expensive, especially compared to the cost of obtaining the equivalent nutrients from ordinary foods?
11. Is it a recent discovery that is not available from any other source?
12. Are the claims too good to be true, or does it promise the impossible?

Take these questions into consideration the next time you are looking for that nutritional edge to enhance your performance. Not all nutritional supplements are useless, but a good majority of them do not provide any more benefit than eating the right foods at the right times. There are products that may help you become a better athlete, but you must do your research first to make sure the product is safe and legal and that it actually holds true to the claims that it is making.

If you decide to take a nutrition supplement, I recommend selecting those that meet the following minimum criteria:

- Carry USP (United States Pharmacopoeia) on the label. "USP" on the label means that the supplement passes tests for dissolution (how well it dissolves), disintegration, potency, and purity. The manufacturer should also be able to demonstrate that the product passes tests for content potency, purity, and uniformity.
- Made by nationally known food and drug manufacturers. Reputable manufacturers follow strict quality control procedures. I have often called supplement companies for athletes to ask about their quality control methods, and company representatives have hung up on me or not provided any

information at all. If this happens to you, your coach, or sport dietitian, or if the company does this or does not answer questions or address complaints, simply do not use their product. It is not worth the risk.

- Supported by research. Reputable companies should provide research from peer-reviewed scientific journals to support claims. If not listed on their supplement or Web site, feel free to call their customer service department and ask for clinical research. If they do not know what you are talking about or state that there is no research, that should raise a red flag, and you should cross their supplement off your "to use" list.

- Accurate and appropriate claims. If statements are unclear or the label makes preposterous claims, it is unlikely that the company follows good quality control procedures. If the claims sound too good to be true, they probably are.

There you have it. Do your research and take your time when choosing supplements, and remember, athlete beware!

NUTRITION SUPPLEMENTS FOR ATHLETES

There are a tremendous number of nutrition supplements on the market that claim to improve performance in some way, shape, or form. And, as I mentioned earlier, all athletes take a supplement at some point throughout their training and competition year. How can I be so certain of this fact? It's simple: I separate supplements into three categories for athletes to help them better understand the function of the supplement and also increase awareness of why they should or should not take a supplement. Of these three categories, I guarantee that you take one product or another at some point throughout your year. The following represents the three classes that I use to teach athletes about supplements:

1. Dietary: micronutrients such as calcium, iron, zinc, and multivitamins. Used for certain vitamin and mineral deficiencies.

2. Sports: energy bars, gels, sports drinks, and electrolyte supplements. Their primary use is before, during, and after training.

3. Ergogenic: antioxidants, amino acids, creatine, caffeine, sodium bicarbonate, energy drinks with the extra ingredients added for mental focus or energy production, adaptogens, androstendione, beta-hydroxy-beta-methylbutyrate (HMB), carnitine, conjugated linoleic acid (CLA), glucosamine/chondroitin, chromium picolinate, dehydroepiandrosterone (DHEA), glutamine, medium-chain triglycerides (MCT), pyruvate, glycerol, bicarbonate, ginseng, coenzyme Q-10, arginine/lysine/ornithine, branched-chain amino acids, niacin. Carbohydrates and fluid are also classified as ergogenic aids, but they were already discussed in Chapter 3.

Of these three categories, ergogenic aids are usually the most popular among athletes because they are thought of more as having a direct impact on performance. Although the other two categories certainly contribute to improving performance, they are not as "sexy" as the ergogenic aids category. Even though this certainly is not meant to be an all-inclusive review, I highlight the most commonly used nutrition supplements used by most endurance, strength, power, combat, acrobat, and team sport athletes. Do not be alarmed if you do not find a supplement that you were thinking about taking or are currently taking. The nutrition supplement market is ever-changing, and I am merely highlighting the more popular ones that athletes normally take.

Dietary

Calcium

Calcium is the most abundant mineral in the body and accounts for about 40% of total mineral stores for most healthy, adult athletes. Ninety-nine percent of calcium is present in the bones and teeth, with the remaining stores used for muscular contractions and metabolic functions, such as activating enzymes that break down muscle glycogen for energy production.

To understand the reason that some athletes choose to supplement with calcium, it is first important to understand how calcium is regulated and excreted. Two hormones (parathyroid and calcitonin) and vitamin D are involved in calcium regulation. The body is very efficient in regulating calcium; thus excessive or poor dietary intakes of calcium rarely result in many changes in calcium levels in the body. However, a deficiency or toxicity of any nutrient does not happen overnight. Any dietary imbalance, coupled with an athlete's demanding training schedule, can result in calcium alterations over time, which is why it is important to pay particular attention to your overall dietary calcium intake on a daily basis.

When your blood calcium levels decrease, parathyroid hormone is released and increases the activation of vitamin D in the kidneys, which act to decrease the amount of calcium lost in the urine. In addition, vitamin D increases the absorption of calcium from the small intestine and resorption from your bones. Your body is fine-tuned to ensure that calcium remains in balance to support its needs.

However, some athletes may not consume enough dietary calcium. Athletes competing in weight-class or aesthetic sports in which calorie restriction is popular may fall into this category. In addition, eating fewer calcium-rich foods during childhood could result in poor calcium deposition and could lead to bone deformities; if this practice is continued, peak bone mass may be lower, which could increase the risk of osteoporosis. Having a low calcium intake during your early developmental years is only the beginning. If you continue to eat low amounts of calcium as an adult, this can lead to excessive calcium resorption from the bone, which increases your risk of osteomalacia. This condition increases your risk for bone fractures.

With some exceptions, it is possible to acquire all of your calcium needs through food. As mentioned previously, if you compete in a sport that involves calorie restriction for weight-cutting, aesthetic-judging, or lower body weights for better economy (or if you simply do not eat calcium-rich foods), it may be impossible to consume enough calcium. Because of calcium's role in exercise, muscular contraction, efficient hormone and neuro-transmitter activity, and effective blood clotting, many athletes justify the use of a calcium supplement.

Intakes of calcium may be higher for athletes than non-athletes because calcium is lost in sweat. It is recommended to consume between 1,300–1,500 milligrams of calcium per day (normal rec-ommendations are 1,000 milligrams per day). The tolerable upper intake level (UL) per day is 2,500 milligrams. Toxicity symptoms over the UL include constipation, kidney stones, cardiac arrhyth-mia, and malabsorption of iron, magnesium, and zinc, so do not consume more than this daily amount.

Female athletes who restrict their caloric intake and become very lean can become amenorrheic. Amenorrhea is strongly associated with poor bone development in young athletes or bone demineralization in older athletes. Without the production of estrogen, they can lose a great deal of calcium. Even if an amen-orrheic athlete consumes enough calcium, this is not enough to maintain or develop healthy bones, because the combination of low estrogen and amenorrhea inhibits normal bone development or maintenance. It is critical for these athletes to increase their calorie intake, with special emphasis on consuming calcium (but not over the UL).

FUELSTORY #1

Many calcium supplements are available to athletes, and one in par-ticular, Viactiv, has quite an appealing taste. It is a caramel-like chew that comes in many different flavors. I remember hearing from one of my sport dietitian colleagues who worked with a collegiate female gymnastic team that the abuse of this particular supplement was widespread. In fact, she told me that many of the athletes restrict their daily calories but eat an entire canister of these calcium chews in one day. One canister contained 30,000 milligrams of calcium and 1,200 calories.

For other athletes, calcium supplementation may not be necessary because the mineral is found in many foods, including dairy products, fortified foods such as soy milk and orange juice, and dark green, leafy vegetables and legumes.

Iron

Iron, one of the most abundant minerals on earth, is a component of hemoglogin, the protein found in red blood cells, which carry oxygen to your cells, and myoglobin, the protein found in heart and skeletal muscle, which carries oxygen to those muscles. Iron is also a component of certain oxidative enzymes that are needed to form energy in your body. The recommended intake of iron is about 10 times the estimated average daily loss because of the low absorption rate of iron in the body. The daily recommended intake does not account for iron that is lost as the result of a high training load followed by athletes. There are different stages associated with iron deficiencies, which are explained in the following:

Stage 1: Diminished total body iron. Identified by a reduction of serum ferritin.

Stage 2: Reduced red blood cell formation. This happens when your iron supply is not able to support new red blood cell production. High levels of zinc protoporphryin (ZPP) can indicate this stage, because, when iron is not available, zinc is used in its place and forms ZPP.

Stage 3: Iron deficiency anemia. Hemoglobin concentration drops below the normal range.

Some athletes, particularly menstruating female and vegetarian athletes, distance runners, and those on calorie-restricted diets (common in weight-class and/or aesthetic sports), are more prone to iron deficiency anemia (discussed in more detail in Chapter 6). However, it is important to remember that any athlete can be prone to iron deficiencies. I have personally seen low iron stores in male football and tennis players, swimmers and gymnasts, track and field athletes, cross-country runners, triathletes, and in female basketball players. Maintaining iron balance and getting enough iron in your body can be difficult, because iron is lost through sweat, urine, the GI tract, and foot-strike hemolysis. If an athlete has low iron stores, the body's ability to make red blood cells is limited, which leads to a decrease in the oxygen-carrying capacity of the blood. Because athletes depend on oxygen delivery to working muscles, even a slight imbalance of iron stores can have significant effects on performance.

The main symptom of iron deficiency anemia is fatigue that worsens with exertion. Fatigue is common and can have many different causes (such as other nutritional imbalances, illness, or stress). If you experience normal fatigue throughout the day and it is not worsened with exercise, the cause is likely not iron deficiency by itself. However, other signs of iron deficiency anemia are a decrease in performance, sleepiness and abnormal fatigue, poor concentration, moodiness or irritability, and always feeling cold.

Iron overload, although not as common as iron deficiency, can occur with excessive supplementation or in athletes who are susceptible to the genetic disease, hemochromatosis. Hemachromatosis affects about 2–3 out of 1,000 individuals and is caused by exces-

---

FUELTIP

Many athletes are aware that one of the telltale signs of iron deficiency is fatigue upon physical exertion. In more than one instance, when I have asked athletes why they are taking iron, they state that it is to improve their energy levels. Even though it is true that iron is a component of oxidative enzymes that yield energy, iron is not a direct energy source itself. In fact, because of serious health consequences and the pro-oxidant effects of consuming too much iron supplement, it is only recommended to supplement with iron after having a blood analysis done and consulting a sport dietitian and/or sport physician who specializes in working with athletes. Normal ranges of iron differ from athletes to non athletes, and the values often seen in lab analyses do not account for values that are specific to the athlete, gender, and sport.

sive storage of iron in the body, which can lead to cirrhosis of the liver, heart failure, and possibly death.

Intense exercise may increase the need for iron by 30%. This may be as a result of increased red blood cell turnover, effects of increased nitric oxide, or other unknown mechanisms. In sports, especially in endurance, weight-class, and aesthetic sports, where low body weight can be an advantage, caloric restriction can result in inadequate dietary iron intake. However, the most common cause of a low hematocrit (a ratio of red blood cells to whole blood cells) in athletes is dilutional pseudo-anemia, which is a dilution of the blood caused by plasma expansion in the beginning of a training program. Although the actual number of red blood cells is not decreased, serum ferritin is affected and is often misdiagnosed by health practitioners. It is important to discuss your training program with healthcare personnel in order to provide them with information regarding your training cycle.

A number of clinical markers describe iron status, including serum iron, red blood cell count, hemoglobin, hematocrit, total iron-binding capacity, and serum ferritin. Serum ferritin, a marker of stored iron, is not tapped into until levels of iron become too low to support demands. For example, if your body is using and excreting more iron than it is receiving from food, the ferritin level slowly declines.

FUELTIP

Replenishment of iron stores, or a positive trend to getting back to "normal," typically takes about 6–8 weeks. Supplementing with iron has not been found to improve performance in athletes who are not deficient. If you use an iron supplement under direction from a sport dietitian and/or sport physician, be sure to have your hemoglobin and serum ferritin, hemoglobin, and hematocrit levels checked regularly, about 2–4 times per year, to prevent complications from iron overload. The dosage is prescribed by your health professional.

Lastly, if you are traveling to a high altitude (>5,000 feet) for an extended period, you may have to increase your iron intake temporarily through food and possibly supplementation, because, under these conditions, your body increases the production of red blood cells, which tap into your iron stores.

Zinc

Zinc is a component of many enzymes in the body and is involved in many functions: most notably for an athlete, protein synthesis, immune function, and DNA synthesis. Zinc is also a necessary component for an enzyme, lactate dehydrogenase (LDH), which is important for rapid synthesis of energy from carbohydrates. Enhanced LDH activity could be beneficial to athletes involved in strength- and power-based sports that require a high amount of energy for a short time.

As good as this may sound, the hard truth is that zinc and athletic performance have not been thoroughly investigated in research, and current scientific research does not support taking zinc as a stand-alone supplement. Chronically high zinc intakes in athletes have not been researched or tested in terms of their effects and safety. In fact, zinc toxicity can result in imbalances of other nutrients, specifically copper, and as little as 3–10 times the recommended dietary intake of zinc reduces copper absorption.

FUELTIP

Zinc is easily found in many foods, including meat, poultry, fish, eggs, shellfish, nuts, vegetables, and whole grains. Because copper status, in particular, can be significantly compromised with zinc supplementation, it is not recommended for healthy athletes without a clinical zinc deficiency to take zinc independent of a basic multi-vitamin.

Multi-vitamins

Whether or not to take a daily multi-vitamin has always been a hot topic among athletes, and it is not an easy question to answer. I often periodize multi-vitamin use throughout the annual training year, based on high and low training loads, travel, past immunosuppression rates, and possible deficiencies.

There are many reasons to take a multi-vitamin, and it is generally thought that athletes engaging in strenuous and/or long-duration training may have increased needs for some vitamins and minerals (especially depending on their current daily dietary pattern). What is not known exactly—and thus no specific recommendations can be made—is which vitamins and minerals are needed in excess by some athletes. Generally speaking, I firmly believe it to be good practice for some athletes to take a multi-vitamin to meet their expenditure needs, which are associated with their gender and possible micronutrient deficiencies.

Sports Supplements

Energy bars

There is quite a variety of energy bars on the market, ranging from low-calorie and low-carbohydrate bars to meal-replacement bars. There are some significant differences among them besides the obvious variations in calories, carbohydrate, protein, and fat content. You should be aware of these differences before choosing a bar. However, you only know this if you read the fine print found in a not-so-convenient location on the wrapper. I am referring to the ingredients list.

How many times do you read the nutrition facts label but not the ingredients list? I am guessing that this happens quite often. I urge you to read the ingredients list before making the final decision to choose an energy bar. Why? Because some of the ingredients are not healthy and can actually impair your performance!

Here is a list of some of the more popular ingredients found in energy bars. Remember that ingredients are listed on the label in order of their presence; this means that any ingredient listed in the top three is present in large quantities.

Fractionated Palm Kernel Oil

Palm kernel oil is predominantly a saturated fat. When the palm oil is fractionated, it has a higher concentration of saturated fat than regular palm oil. In this form, it is used for the convenience of manufacturers for its stability and melting characteristics. Be aware that fractionated palm kernel oil is used in many energy bars, usually found in the coating or icing.

Glycerin (Glycerine, Glycerol)

Glycerin, a commercial product that's principal component is glycerol, is not technically a carbohydrate, although it does contain about the same number of calories per gram. Glycerin is a type of alcohol that is one of the by-products of fat metabolism. The interesting thing about glycerin in some energy bars is that manufacturers include it but do not count its contribution to calorie and carbohydrate totals on the label. What this means is that there may be more carbohydrates and calories than stated. One energy bar that the manufacturer stated contained only 2 grams of carbohydrate was tested by ConsumberLab.com and was found to have 20 additional grams of carbohydrate from glycerin. Quite a significant difference! My recommendation for you is to minimize its use because all of the calories may not be reported on the labels of products that contain glycerin.

Green Tea Extract

Green tea is associated with a mild increase in thermogenesis, which means that it increases the amount of calories that you burn. This is mostly a result of its caffeine content, and it is relatively safe to consume. However, if an energy bar contains green tea extract and it does in fact increase the amount of calories that you burn, this bar is not beneficial to eat during exercise because some non weight-class athletes have a hard enough time trying to replenish the calories that they burn during training.

Fiber

Fiber content in grams is always reported on the nutrition facts label. As you know, fiber is a very healthy nutrient that is a necessity in your normal eating program. However, when present in larger amounts, it could cause more bathroom breaks than you want to take during training and, for some athletes, could be a huge burden during a competition.

OTHER THINGS TO CONSIDER

It is said that knowledge is power. I believe this statement is true, because increasing your knowledge about the less popular ingredients in energy bars allows you to have more power in choosing the right energy bar for your body and training.

Also, don't forget to look at the very fine print on energy bar labels stating whether the product was manufactured on equipment that processes nuts, wheat, and seeds or may contain peanuts or traces of other nuts. If you are allergic to nuts or seeds or are sensitive to gluten (wheat), avoid bars with these warnings.

Energy gels

Energy gels are a mix between a sports drink and an energy bar. The primary purpose of energy gels is to provide carbohydrates that can be used for immediate use to fuel working muscles. Unfortunately, many manufacturers of energy gels believe that more is better and they add nutrients that are simply not necessary during exercise. They usually extrapolate from one or two nutrient success stories to believe that the addition of nutrients benefits the entire gel.

It is important to consider the type(s) of sugar that the energy gel uses to determine whether it is the type that you want during training or competition. Your body is different from that of your competitors or teammates, and it may not process a certain type of sugar in the same way that it does for someone else. Also keep in mind that energy gels have roughly a 55–65% carbohydrate concentration (compared to 4–8% in most sports drinks), which makes it a bit tougher to digest during training and competition. Adequate water must be consumed with an energy gel.

Sports Drinks

There are so many categories of sports drinks these days that choosing one to meet your performance needs is very confusing. There are products that have been around for 30 or more years and products that have only been introduced in the last few years. Aside from what I term the "frill ingredients" (i.e., vitamins, minerals, and herbs), the main differences among these drinks include the types of sugar, concentration of carbohydrates, the osmolality, and the sodium content. Here is a bit more information about each:

1. Type(s) of sugar

   The most common include sucrose, glucose, and fructose. The type of sugar affects sweetness. Sweetness can reduce fluid intake. High fructose levels can cause GI distress. Fairly new research indicates that the combination of sugars (specifically glucose or maltodextrin and fructose) increases carbohydrate absorption because the two sugars utilize different transport mechanisms across the small intestine. Using more than one type of carbohydrate source also allows manufacturers to use various textures and taste combinations.

2. Carbohydrate concentration

   Research has shown that a sports drink with 6–8% carbohydrate concentration is well absorbed and utilized by the body for energy. Anything above 8% delays emptying from the stomach and could cause stomach problems during your training session or competition. There are drinks that contain less than 6% and work well for some athletes.

3. Osmolality

   Osmolality is a term referring to the number of particles in a solution. A solution with fewer particles (low osmolality) tends to produce faster fluid absorption. High osmolality (>400) can slow fluid absorption. Most mainstream sports drinks have an osmolality between 280–360, but certainly not all do.

4. Sodium

I have personally worked with many athletes who redefine normal sodium losses during training. Because of this, I promote more sodium for athletes competing in the following situations:

a. Longer than two hours

b. Hot and humid environment

c. High sweat rate

d. High sweat sodium concentration

The body regulates sodium concentration very well, and it is extremely difficult to consume too much without your body triggering your brain to consume more water in an effort to balance out the higher sodium content. It is difficult to recommend sodium levels to athletes because needs differ. In addition, many athletes find additional methods of supplementing sodium, such as eating pretzels, crackers, energy bars or gels, and using salt tablets/powders. For this reason, I do not offer a minimum sodium amount for sports drinks. Rather, as discussed in Chapter 3, I recommend a total amount of sodium to be consumed during training or competition. It is important for your sports drink to include some sodium because it enhances taste, optimizes absorption, and maintains fluid balance more effectively.

If you are wondering about vitamins and minerals added to sports drinks, don't spend too much time analyzing the issue. No data exist to show physiological benefits of adding any vitamins to a sports drink. In fact, some B vitamins adversely affect the taste of a beverage and could actually decrease the amount you drink.

The sports drink section always includes protein. The addition of protein to sports drinks has not been without controversy. It has been suggested that consuming a protein-carbohydrate mixture during exercise raises blood insulin to higher levels than carbohydrate alone. Having a higher blood insulin level increases the body's use of carbohydrate in muscle and better delays fatigue. The hormone insulin is responsible for transporting carbohydrate from the blood into the muscle cell, where it can be used for energy.

Research has shown that consuming carbohydrate during exercise delays fatigue by increasing the amount of energy that is supplied by blood glucose, thereby slowing the rate of muscle glycogen depletion. During long exercise sessions of more than 90 minutes, if carbohydrate is in short supply, protein can contribute up to 15% of total energy, but if you are replenishing your carbohydrate stores at consistent intervals, protein use is minimal. A few research studies have shown that the consumption of protein during training can provide additional benefits. These benefits include the following:

- A stronger insulin response. Some research has shown that a small amount of protein added to carbohydrates results in a stronger insulin response, which allows glucose to be delivered to the muscles faster. This, in turn, conserves stored muscle glycogen that can be used at a later time and may delay fatigue.

- Reduced muscle protein breakdown. As mentioned earlier, in longer training sessions of 90 minutes or more, protein can be used as an energy source if carbohydrates are not being constantly replenished. The protein that is used as energy comes from muscle proteins, which means your muscles are breaking down to a certain extent to provide your body with the energy to keep exercising.

- Reduced muscle soreness and damage. New research indicates that consuming protein during a training session or competition can lessen the degree of muscle soreness and damage following the workout, which has benefit for athletes competing in multiple daily training sessions or competing often.

Although the benefits of protein seem to be positive, different responses may occur with the addition of protein. I recommend that if you want to try adding protein during competition, do so in training first. Some athletes I have worked with swear by it; others have experienced stomach problems.

Electrolyte Supplements

There are as many viewpoints on taking electrolyte supplements as there are training programs. Electrolyte supplements typically include plain salt tablets, capsules, powders, fluids, and strips. There are also full-spectrum electrolyte supplements that offer additional electrolytes, including calcium, magnesium, and potassium. The basis for including more minerals in electrolyte supplements is mainly because of what is lost in sweat. Many compounds are found in sweat, including ammonia, copper, creatinine, iodine, iron, lactic acid, manganese, phosphorus, urea, uric acid, sodium, chloride, calcium, potassium, and magnesium. The last five are the micronutrients that are found in higher quantity in sweat; thus electrolyte supplements containing them boast an ability to replace what is lost as you exercise.

For athletes who have a high sweat rate and sodium concentration and train in a hot and humid environment, additional electrolyte supplements are needed, regardless of the type. It is unrealistic for any sports drink on the market to supply the necessary quantities of electrolytes for these athletes. I have seen laboratory tested sweat sodium concentrations exceed 3,000 milligrams per hour; the highest I have witnessed were from an elite, male mountain bike athlete, who topped the scales at losing more than

---

FUELSTORY #2

Electrolyte supplementation is not sport-specific. I have worked with football players, triathletes, baseball players, tennis players, sailors, cross-country athletes, marathoners, motocross racers, and swimmers who have all required extra electrolytes during training and competition. Remember, if you are a heavy sweater and live/train/compete in hot and/or humid conditions, you need to rely on an electrolyte supplement. When choosing one, make sure that it has at least 200 milligrams of sodium per serving.

5,000 milligrams per hour. As you can see, for these athletes, who are very much on the extreme side of sodium loss, electrolyte supplementation is crucial for their success in maintaining fluid balance and preventing hyponatremia. Athletes who have a more normal sweat sodium loss per hour typically lose between 700–1,200 milligrams of sodium.

Ergogenic Aids

Adaptogens

Adaptogens have been a fairly new inclusion to the nutrition supplement market, although they have existed for thousands of years. An adaptogen is a substance that increases resistance to physical and emotional stress, stress-related imbalances, and environmental pollution. Some also contain polysaccharides, which have been reported to stimulate the immune system, which works in a synergistic way to increase the body's ability to fight illness before it hits. Some common examples of adaptogens include ginseng, ashwagandha, schisandra, rhodiola, cordyceps, reishi, and maitake.

One of the major actions of adaptogens relative to athletes is their ability to increase resistance to the catabolic effects of high-intensity training. This in itself caters to all categories of sports and athletes during higher training loads.

As the intensity of training increases, it forces your body to use its natural defense mechanisms to help repair and replace the damage that happens. Using adaptogens could allow this defense mechanism to work more efficiently, thus allowing you to train at a higher level.

It is likely more beneficial to take adaptogens throughout the more intense training cycles, and most of the current research has targeted physiological markers that are important to athletes, such as VO_{2peak}, pulmonary ventilation and time to exhaustion, and others, such as creatine kinase and C-reactive protein activity, that are important to all athletes. Some recent research has shown a link to prevention of overtraining syndrome, providing protective effects from inflammation and infection, increasing fat utilization, and slowing glycogen utilization.

Most adaptogens are not conventional compounds, but consist mostly of herbs. There are minimal effects or concerns of toxicity by taking in too much, but, as with any supplement, the risk of abuse exists. In addition, there may be accompanying side effects of taking herbal remedies, so it is wise to check with a health professional who is well informed about these types of supplements prior to taking them.

Because of the wide array of adaptogens on the market, strength, power, endurance, and team sport athletes could benefit from taking them—during their higher-volume and intensity training throughout their competitive year—or athletes resuming training after an off-season, unplanned break, or the beginning of a new sport.

Amino Acids

Amino acids are the building blocks of protein and can serve as an energy source for skeletal muscle, and protein synthesis can occur at rest even when essential amino acids are consumed in relatively small amounts (15 grams).

Branched-chain amino acids (BCAAs) are becoming more popular among athletes because of their many possible performance benefits. These essential amino acids are comprised of the amino acids leucine, isoleucine, and valine. They can be oxidized by the skeletal muscle to provide the muscles with energy, enhance post-exercise muscle protein synthesis, and reduce exercise-induced muscle damage. The average BCAA content of food proteins is roughly 15% of the total amino acid content; thus athletes consume adequate amounts through food if a well-balanced eating plan is followed. Some athletes may require a higher protein intake, depending on the sport and training cycle, because BCAAs are oxidized in greater amounts during exercise versus at rest. However, the research is not conclusive; there is evidence on either side to support the argument of increased needs versus normal needs obtained through food. What is certain is that athletes must periodize their protein intake based on the physical demands of their training. If volumes and intensities fluctuate throughout a year with different endurance and resistance exercise goals, protein intake should match these changes to support physiological adaptations.

Arginine is another amino acid that may be important in regard to exercise training and preventing protein breakdown when combined with BCAAs. When consumed, arginine facilitates the removal of ammonia through the urea cycle, which could reduce fatigue. It is also a precursor for nitric oxide, a potent vasodilator that could enhance athletic performance by improving blood flow to and from working muscles. It also acts as a stimulator of growth hormone and the hormone insulin. During shorter, moderate to intense aerobic exercise, a dose of only 2 grams of BCAAs and arginine before exercise has been shown to suppress the catabolic protein response to exercise, showing that these specific amino acids have a place in an athlete's daily nutrition plan.

Whether or not supplemental amino acids are needed in addition to those found in the daily nutrition plan of athletes still remains debatable, especially considering that many sports nutrition supplements already contain amino acids. It is wise to look at the inclusion of amino acids into your nutrition plan based on energy expenditure levels and training load changes.

Antioxidants

There is a great deal of research on antioxidants and conclusions that span the gamut from worthless to worthwhile. For many years we have known how powerful vitamins E and C, beta-carotene, and selenium are. Recently, a large number of antioxidants, some with names that are virtually impossible to pronounce, have made their way into the athlete marketplace. It seems as if anything can be called an antioxidant, as more and more compounds are being discovered in foods that classify as having health and performance benefits.

You have certainly heard the term before, but do you truly know what antioxidants are and how they function? Antioxidants are compounds that suppress free radicals that inflict harm on the

Table 5.1
Examples of Antioxidants

Water Soluble	Lipid Soluble
Ascorbic Acid (vitamin C)	Alpha-tocopherol (vitamin E)
Glutathione	Ubiquinol (coenzyme Q)
Lipoic Acid	
Uric Acid	

body. To reduce the harmful effects of free radicals, your body has an antioxidant system that includes antioxidant enzymes such as catalase, glutathione peroxidase and superoxide dismutase, and nonenzymatic antioxidants such as vitamins A, C, and E and glutathione (see Table 5.1). When your body's antioxidant defense system is bombarded with increased free radical production, your body is in a higher oxidative stress state. This can be detrimental to your performance because there are positive links to increased inflammation and cell damage and possibly overtraining syndrome.

Free radicals, also known as pro-oxidants, are reactive oxygen or nitrogen species (referred to sometimes as ROS, RNS, or RONS) and are formed during metabolism, immune cell activation, inflammation, and infection as well as other situations and environmental factors (see Table 5.2). Free radicals are highly reactive, unstable molecules that have an unpaired electron in their outer shell and can have positive effects on your immune system

Table 5.2
Environmental Factors and Situations that Contribute ROS/RNS

Carbon and Nitrogen Dioxide (CO_2 and NO_2), Pollutants
UV light
Altitude
Smoking
Radiation
High intensity exercise
Drugs
Inflammation

and metabolic functions and negative effects on lipid, protein, and DNA oxidation. Your body is well equipped to handle free radicals, but if antioxidants are unavailable, or if the free radical production becomes excessive, damage can occur and your body will experience an oxidative stress response.

Free radicals often get a bad rap. Did you know that free radicals are actually produced during exercise and your antioxidant defense system is actually strengthened? However, there is a catch. Exhaustive and/or intense training seem to be the main culprits of turning free radicals from good to bad. If you participate in high-intensity training of any sort, you are subject to a higher free radical production. Oxidative stress is unavoidable for athletes, but of special concern is the oxidative stress due to increased oxygen consumption during exercise. This is in addition to a higher exposure to environmental oxidative stress from altitude, ultraviolet rays, inflammation from muscle damage, and pollution. Being an athlete increases your exposure to situations that can increase oxidative stress.

Although many scientists and athletes like to argue the point, it is still not clear from all of the research on antioxidants and athletes whether or not higher-intensity exercise increases the need for additional antioxidants. What is agreed upon by experts of all types is that antioxidants obtained from food sources often have a higher bioavailability. This does not mean antioxidants in supplement form are not beneficial. It is sometimes the opposite, depending on an athlete's normal eating habits. Antioxidants such as vitamins A, C, and E, vitamin-like compounds such as glutathione and lipoic acid, and phytochemicals such as flavonoids and polyphenols, have a significant role in improving the body's defense system whether consumed through foods or as dietary supplements.

There is a system that measures the quality of antioxidants that is extremely useful when choosing blueberries or bananas at the grocery store. The oxygen reactive absorbency capacity (ORAC) is a quantitative measure of an antioxidant's ability to neutralize oxygen free radicals. The clinical data supporting this methodology has become the gold standard for the measurement of an antioxidant's free radical–scavenging ability. Foods that score high help protect cells and their components from oxidative damage. The higher a food's ORAC score, the better it is at helping our bodies fight the damages of oxidative stress.

The ORAC score covers all the antioxidants in foods. Antioxidants cannot easily be measured separately, but the ORAC score test can identify which nutrients are the important antioxidants. Combinations of nutrients found in foods may have greater protective benefits than each nutrient on its own. I honestly do not know many athletes who do not take some type of antioxidant supplement to try to obtain their daily nutrients, and while there is certainly nothing wrong with this, this method cannot and should not replace eating foods rich in antioxidants.

The National Institute on Aging developed the ORAC method, and the U.S. Department of Agriculture and Brunswick Labs have been instrumental in perfecting the ORAC assay procedure and testing various foods to determine ORAC levels.

Specific to food, different types of fruits and vegetables have different ORAC scores. The U.S. Department of Agriculture (USDA) recommends that individuals consume between 3,000 and 5,000 ORAC units per day. This is for the non-athlete, and as oxidative stress increases due to training, environmental factors, and other situations, I recommend athletes push the 5,000 mark and try to consume more around 7,000–10,000 ORAC units per day. Refer to Table 5.3 for high–ORAC level, antioxidant-rich foods.

Studies have shown that eating foods with high ORAC scores will raise the antioxidant levels in the blood by 10–25%. Many experts recommend eating around 5,000 units per day to have a significant effect on antioxidant levels. You can use the information in Table 5.3 to help attain this level, but for athletes, eating five servings of fruits and vegetables just doesn't cut it in the quest to reduce oxidative stress. I often recommend eating at least 8–10 servings of brightly colored fruits and vegetables to begin to help quench the free radicals that you are producing during training and under certain environmental conditions. I know this may

Table 5.3
ORAC Levels of Antioxidant-Rich Foods (Serving size is approximately 3.5 ounces.)

Fruits	ORAC Level	Vegetables	ORAC level	Other Food	ORAC Level
Prunes	5,770	Garlic	1,939	Unprocessed cacao powder	26,000
Pomegranates	3,307	Kale	1,770	Dark chocolate	13,120
Raisins	2,830	Spinach	1,260	Milk chocolate	6,740
Blueberries	2,400	Yellow squash	1,150	Tofu	205
Blackberries	2,036	Brussels sprouts	980		
Cranberries	1,750	Alfalfa sprouts	930		
Strawberries	1,540	Broccoli flowers	890		
Raspberries	1,220	Beets	840		
Plums	949	Red bell pepper	710		
Oranges	750	Kidney beans	460		
Red grapes	739	Onion	450		
Cherries	670	Corn	400		
Kiwi	602	Eggplant	390		
Pink grapefruit	483	Sweet potato	295		
Banana	210	Cabbage	295		
Apple	207	Carrot	200		

sound unattainable, but if you do the math, it is easier than you think. Sure, if you only eat one or two times per day it will be a challenge, but if you are a frequent eater and average four to eight "feedings" on a daily basis, obtaining the necessary servings of high–ORAC level foods is simple. Add some fruit to a smoothie in the morning and get a couple of servings. Have a moderate-sized salad to accompany your lunch to add a few more ORAC units. Choose fruits and veggies to include in your snacks, and don't forget the vegetables at dinner. Voila! You just achieved at least seven servings without blinking an eye.

FUELTIP

Exercise can increase oxygen utilization from 10 to 20 times over the resting state. With this comes an increase in free radicals—but how effectively can athletes defend against the increased free radicals resulting from exercise? And more importantly, do you need to take extra antioxidants to account for this?

As I mentioned previously, exercise enhances the antioxidant defense system and protects against exercise-induced free radical damage. This proves just how complex the body is as it adapts to the demands of training.

However, intense exercise in untrained individuals overwhelms the antioxidant defense system, which results in an increase in free radicals and thus oxidative stress. For novice athletes, those coming off of an injury, or recreational athletes who may be more sedentary during the week but exercise vigorously on the weekends, there can be more oxidative stress. During these instances, fruits and vegetables become very important in the daily eating programs, as can using a dietary supplement to try to counteract free radical production.

It has been known for some time that vitamin deficiencies can create challenges in training and recovery, and thus the role of antioxidant supplementation in a well-nourished athlete remains controversial. In general, antioxidant supplements have not been shown to be useful as direct performance enhancers.

Although there is little doubt that antioxidants are a necessary component for good health, the debate will continue, regarding whether athletes should take antioxidant supplements to improve performance. Of course, you can generalize that if they promote health, they will also promote a higher level of performance, as it is difficult to perform well without having good health.

And do not fall prey to the philosophy that "If one is good, two must be better." There is increasing knowledge about the toxicity of certain nutrients. For example, in the normal concentrations found in the body, vitamin C and beta-carotene are antioxidants, but at higher concentrations they are actually pro-oxidants.

Include an abundant amount of fruits and vegetables (see Table 5.4) in your eating program, first and foremost. There is certainly nothing wrong with using a dietary supplement as long as you know it is safe, legal, and efficacious. But recall my last point, that taking megadoses of some antioxidants can cause them to contribute more to your body's oxidative stress rather than working against it—so choose your supplement carefully.

Table 5.4
List of Vitamin C, E, Beta-Carotene, Lycopene, and Lutein–Rich Foods

Vitamin C–rich foods	Vitamin E–rich foods	Beta carotene, lycopene, and lutein–rich foods
Orange, orange juice	Almonds	Tomatoes
Cantaloupe	Hazelnuts	Sweet potatoes
Cranberry juice	Sunflower seeds	Carrots
Grapefruit, grapefruit juice	Spinach	Broccoli
Strawberry	Sweet potato	Brussels sprout
Kiwi	Olive, sunflower, canola oils	Spinach
Papaya	Wheat germ	Kale
Spinach	Fortified cereals	Collard greens
Broccoli	Fish oils	Cantaloupe
Sweet red peppers		Mango
Asparagus		Egg yolk

It is estimated that only 10% of the U.S. population consumes five servings of fruits and vegetables per day. Due to the nature of training stressors, athletes may need further protection from the damage of oxidative stress. Some of the newest clinical research suggests that this oxidative protection may even lead to improved performance. With abundant formulas and antioxidant concoctions in the marketplace, do not rely on a single compound. Look for a formula or multi-vitamin that contains a variety of antioxidants. If you are shopping for antioxidant supplements, consider vitamins such as C and E, and beta-carotene, as well other antioxidants such as alpha-lipoic acid and

N-acetylcysteine, which function as glutathione precursors. Also consider the following in your search for an appropriate formula: grape seed extract, carotenoids, pycnogenol, lutein, lycopene, bioflavanoids, green tea, turmeric, and quercetin. In some newer formulas, you can also specifically find antioxidants that have been analyzed for their ORAC value.

The damaging effects of oxidation can take years, even a lifetime, to reveal their impact. Antioxidants should be viewed as insurance against this damage. With long-term consumption of antioxidants, you will support healthy cells, leading to healthy cellular respiration. If you train heavily day in and day out, antioxidants should be a staple in your eating program. With a few months of increased consumption, you should notice reduced incidence of infection, faster recovery, and better workouts.

Beta-Alanine

Beta-alanine has some exciting scientific support behind it and seems promising in its use with athletes. This non-essential amino acid is part of the amino acid carnosine and is needed to continually replenish the body's stores of carnosine to fuel high-intensity exercise. Carnosine is a potent buffer of hydrogen ions and increased amounts of this amino acid has direct correlation with improved anaerobic and aerobic performance, which would be useful for just about every athlete, from weightlifters to triathletes. Muscle carnosine synthesis is limited by the availability of beta-alanine thus by supplementing with beta-alanine, there would be an increase in carnosine stores, which could then provide more of a buffering mechanism during exercise.

Consistent, high-intensity exercise increases the amount of muscle carnosine, but research has shown that taking a daily beta-alanine supplement increases carnosine levels more than training and eating carnosine-rich foods (mostly meat products). Beta-alanine, through its effect on carnosine, can also synthesize lactic acid to be reused as fuel and can generate nitric oxide synthase, which makes the vasodilator nitric oxide. This could be an additional benefit to some athletes, as an increase in blood flow delivers more nutrients to the muscles.

Research has been done on strength and power athletes and endurance athletes, and as with most research, there are some studies that show results and others that do not. But the consensus is that supplemental beta-alanine can increase carnosine levels, which can have a positive effect in delaying neuromuscular fatigue, using lactic acid as fuel, improve intra- and extracellular buffering capabilities, total work completed, and increased time to exhaustion. There is a harmless side effect of beta-alanine supplementation: about half of the athletes who take it will experience parathesia, a tingling sensation in the upper extremities resulting from beta-alanine's actions as a neurotransmitter. Current research indicates that a daily dose ranging from 3 to 6 grams is sufficient to raise carnosine stores.

Beta-hydroxy-beta-methylbutyrate (HMB)

HMB is a byproduct of the amino acid leucine in the body. Approximately 5–10% of leucine is metabolized into HMB, and about 0.2–0.4 grams of HMB are made in the body per day, depending on how much leucine you consume. This supplement has been used predominantly in strength, power, and aesthetic sport athletes as a method of improving lean muscle mass and reducing body fat. However, some endurance athletes have turned to it specifically for its claim of reducing muscle breakdown after exercise.

While the exact mechanisms of HMB's action are not known, it is theorized that it may inhibit or slow the breakdown of muscle during higher-intensity exercise. This sounds extremely beneficial to a wide array of athletes, but current research simply does not support the claims that are made about using HMB.

While there are no reported adverse effects or safety concerns at this time, regarding the use of HMB, the research does not seem to support the claims one hundred percent of the time. Additionally, because HMB can be made via the amino acid leucine, and due to the fact that leucine is obtained by eating animal products, it is not beneficial for athletes to use this supplement as an ergogenic aid.

Caffeine

Caffeine, the most widely consumed drug in the world, is one of the most researched and ergogenic aids in terms of athletic performance. The ability of caffeine to enhance muscular work has existed since the early 1900s. Most of the research in caffeine supports an ergogenic benefit in endurance athletes, but the data has been conflicting with strength and power athletes.

Caffeine acts on the central nervous system (CNS) as a stimulant by increasing the release of adrenaline, which can improve mental alertness, using body fat as fuel, and sparing glycogen at lower- to moderate-intensity exercise. In higher-intensity exercise, caffeine has been shown to decrease the rating of perceived exertion, increase carbohydrate oxidation when consumed with a carbohydrate source, and allow athletes to reach higher levels of lactate. Caffeine can also improve cardiac efficiency by opening up the bronchioles (smaller airways that are responsible for sending oxygen to the lungs to be absorbed and sent throughout the body).

Caffeine is often mistakenly classified as a diuretic (causing loss of water from the body). However, recent research suggests that over a 24-hour period, caffeine does not exhibit a dehydrating effect on the body. Moderate amounts of caffeine can be consumed throughout the day as long as other beverages are consumed to aid in positive fluid balance. It is important to remember that caffeine has a half-life of 4–6 hours, which means that roughly half of the amount ingested will still remain in the body 4–6 hours later.

The practice of discontinuing caffeine prior to a competition has become popular in some athletes because of the habituation response to caffeine. The theory is that the more caffeine you consume on a daily basis (thus becoming habituated to it), the less ergogenic effect you will see with it, because your body is so used to a high amount. Abstaining from the use of caffeine for days or weeks before a competition is thought to allow the body to become accustomed to not having caffeine; then, reintroducing it shortly before competition is thought to cause an ergogenic effect. Whether or not athletes choose to do this is an individual decision. However, I have seen many athletes experience negative side effects when moving from a high daily caffeine dose to a low one. I normally recommend athletes try this a few times in training well before their competition to determine whether there are any negative consequences for them. Additionally, as I will discuss soon, many athletes do not consume a high enough dose of caffeine prior to competitions to create an ergogenic response. Thus, I have seen much success with having athletes simply decrease their daily dose of caffeine by about 50% in the 5–7 days before a competition, and then use clinically significant doses of caffeine prior to competition for the performance-enhancing effects.

As mentioned previously, there is good research proving that caffeine has an ergogenic benefit for endurance athletes. For strength, power, and team-sport athletes, roughly half of the available studies conclude that there is a performance improvement, while the other half does not. Interestingly, the positive effects were seen on more elite athletes who did not regularly consume caffeine on a daily basis.

The protocol that should be used to seek improvement in performance through the use of caffeine includes the following:

- Consume 3–9 milligrams of caffeine per kilogram of body weight, 60–75 minutes before competition.
- If the competition is prolonged, it may be justified to consume 1–3 milligrams of caffeine every 90–120 minutes. More is not better in this scenario, as too high a dose frequently causes GI distress.

Caffeine has been proven to improve performance when used correctly. However, using caffeine as an ergogenic aid should be done with caution due to the higher levels needed to stimulate the central nervous system. Too much caffeine can cause athletes to become anxious, delirious, and irritable; thus it is extremely important that athletes not abuse its use in sport.

Creatine

Creatine, a nitrogenous organic compound, is made from the amino acids glycine, methionine, and arginine. The majority of creatine in the body is found in the skeletal muscle, with a low amount synthesized in the liver, kidneys, and pancreas. It is found in foods such as beef, salmon, tuna, pork, and herring. It is theorized that supplementing with creatine can improve events that last from 90 seconds to 4 minutes, by reducing the body's reliance on anaerobic glycolysis and reducing lactate levels, thus delaying fatigue. This could be of great benefit to strength and power athletes, or anyone engaging in a high-power and hypertrophy-producing strength training program.

As discussed earlier in this book, there are three energy systems in the body. Creatine exhibits its positive effect on the phosphocreatine system. Because this energy system is always the first to respond to exercise, it becomes depleted very quickly (in less than 15 seconds). The benefit of supplementing with creatine is that it can improve the ability to generate more ATP (adenosine triphosphate), which can improve energy supply. This results in better, more forceful muscle contractions, which, when combined with a sound resistance training program, produce an increase in muscle mass.

There have been concerns about using creatine in the heat, and its ability to hinder exercise performance. However, a research review article concluded that using creatine does not decrease an athlete's ability to dissipate heat, nor does it negatively affect the fluid balance state—as long as recommended doses were taken. There is typically associated weight gain seen in athletes when using creatine, so athletes should be careful in using it based on their body weight goals and sport requirements (i.e., weight classes).

There are many different methods of using creatine as a supplement. The traditional method has included a loading phase consisting of taking 20 grams of creatine per day for 5–7 days, after which time a maintenance dose of 3–5 grams per day is followed. Another method is to simply consume 3–5 grams per day without a loading phase. Regardless of the method chosen, creatine supplementation should be customized based on each athlete's needs. Additionally, cycling the use of creatine is important, as there are some indications that using creatine for an extended period may reduce its positive effects. Normal cycling patterns include using creatine for 3–8 weeks and then discontinuing its use for 3–4 weeks. For athletes using creatine surrounding a training session, it is normally recommended to introduce creatine beforehand and then follow with another dose, along with carbohydrate and protein for maximal benefit.

Creatine supplementation has been studied in normal, healthy adults, but not in children under 18 years of age. There is no solid information to suggest that using creatine is unsafe for adults, for short periods, but there is no information regarding the use of creatine in children, or over extended periods of time. Additionally, because of the physiological benefit of creatine in regenerating ATP to improve energy, athletes should not use creatine without making sure that adequate calories are also being consumed on a daily basis. The use of creatine should be justified and used carefully by each athlete.

Energy Drinks

The entire beverage market is booming worldwide. Included in this, and of particular interest to athletes, are energy drinks. These beverages are an offshoot of soft drinks, containing a host of other ingredients. Their claims typically boast "improved energy," "improved mental concentration and alertness," and "improved performance"—and although it sounds promising to the athlete, there isn't much scientific evidence, besides the known effects of caffeine, to support the claims. Some of these drinks are a compilation of many herbal ingredients, caffeine derivates, sugar, or artificial sugars that, very simply, will not do anything for you other than give you a caffeine buzz.

If the energy drink contains sugar, it will provide you energy. Sugar equals calories, and calories will provide the body energy if needed. If a drink contains caffeine, it will serve as a central nervous system stimulant, so you may feel more energized, but this feeling may be short-lived, depending on the dose of caffeine present and the frequency with which you drink it. Of course, if it contains artificial sweeteners and no sugar, you will simply obtain a caffeine "high" from it, as it will not technically provide you with energy to supply your muscles for exercise.

There are much better ways to supply your body with the nutrients it needs to sustain exercise, and if you are in search of the caffeine for the mental stimulation, there are far better products that are not a mishmash of other, unnecessary ingredients. Because of the somewhat unknown effects, ingredients, and doses found in energy drinks, it is not recommended that athletes use these as an ergogenic aid in search of optimal performance.

Glutamine

Glutamine, a nonessential amino acid, is the most abundant amino acid in the body. It can be made in muscle, fat tissue, the lungs, the liver, and the brain. It is found in certain foods, such as cabbage, beets, beef, chicken, fish, beans, vegetables, and dairy products. Glutamine is synthesized in skeletal muscle and in adipose tissue, in addition to the lungs, liver, and brain. Because there is evidence that during high-stress situations glutamine demands exceed glutamine supply, which can have a negative impact on performance and immune function, glutamine is often referred to as a "conditional nonessential amino acid." This suggests that during high training loads, it would be necessary to consume extra glutamine, in addition to what is made in the body.

Because of its role in immune function, glutamine may be very important to athletes who may suffer from overtraining syndrome or who are susceptible to upper respiratory tract infections. Athletes can obtain sufficient amounts of glutamine from food during low to moderate training loads; however, for weight-class or aesthetic sports where the restriction of calories is common practice, for endurance athletes competing in strenuous competitions, or for athletes in a high training load cycle, a greater amount of glutamine may be necessary to support immune function and nitrogen (protein) balance.

For maximum results, pay special attention to supplementing with glutamine immediately following long, exhaustive exercise, to restore to physiological levels at the time of depletion. Athletes who consistently use glutamine through their race season may experience improved recovery, improved nitrogen balance, and reduced incidence of infection.

Athletes who typically use glutamine as a supplement do so during strenuous training sessions or competitions, in combination with a sports drink. Consuming single amino acids can cause imbalances of others amino acids, so it is recommended to combine it with other nutrients, especially carbohydrates. Glutamine supplementation may not directly serve as an ergogenic aid; however, it will function to maintain skeletal muscle and immune function, particularly in the previously mentioned athlete groups and accompanying high-volume and intensity training.

Medium-Chain Triglycerides (MCTs)

Fat is not normally thought of as having ergogenic properties; however, one particular type of fat, because of its different metabolic properties, may just turn your head. MCTs are a type of saturated fat with shorter lengths of carbon molecules, which allow them to possess somewhat different characteristics than their longer-length carbon fat cousins. This physical difference causes MCTs to be digested and metabolized more quickly by the liver, so that they can be converted to energy faster. They also do not need L-carnitine as a transporter to enter the mitochondria, to provide energy.

MCTs act similarly to carbohydrates, which has led to the belief that they could be used as a glycogen-sparing fuel source. Many of the claims for MCTs have included providing quick sources of energy for athletes, sparing lean muscle mass, and mobilizing fat stores for energy—all of which could be extremely beneficial for almost any athlete. In reality, though, endurance athletes would likely get the most benefit from this supplement.

MCTs are found in coconut and palm kernel oils, which are very popular ingredients in food and can often be found in energy bars. Taking large doses of MCTs can cause diarrhea and cramping, so if you plan to using them, be sure to experiment with them long before your competition.

Unfortunately, research has shown mixed results and, interestingly, the positive results found with using MCTs have been in individuals who increased their total calorie intake. Studies in which the calories were matched between carbohydrates, versus MCTs and carbohydrates have not found significant improvements in performance. From a research perspective, there is not much convincing evidence to support using MCTs as an ergogenic aid to improve performance, even though there are anecdotal reports from athletes who have had great success with it.

Sodium Bicarbonate and Citrate

Sodium bicarbonate—baking soda—is an alkaline salt that buffers metabolic acids. In theory, this supplement seems extremely promising for athletes of many sports since it has an effect on high-intensity training. During this type of training, lactic acidosis and an increase in hydrogen ions have been associated with exhaustion. This creates a more acidic environment in the body, which is where sodium bicarbonate comes into the picture. It is thought that using sodium bicarbonate/citrate creates a buffer and increases the alkaline reserves, and helps with the removal of the hydrogen ions, which could delay the onset of fatigue and improve performance.

There has been good research to support the ergogenic benefits of sodium bicarbonate/citrate in exercise lasting from 1 to 7 minutes. It would likely benefit strength and power athletes the most and would work well for short interval-training sessions for endurance athletes. However, there is some data to suggest that longer-duration training, as seen in endurance athletes, could also benefit from this supplement.

The most popular loading protocol for sodium bicarbonate/citrate is to consume 0.3–0.5 grams per kilogram of body weight, along with at least 20 ounces of a carbohydrate electrolyte beverage, 2–3 hours before competition.

Sodium bicarbonate has been shown to produce GI distress in some athletes; thus sodium citrate (a milder form of the supplement) has been used with great success in some athletes in an attempt to reduce GI distress symptoms. For athletes who are prone to GI distress or who experience it when using sodium bicarbonate, sodium citrate would be a viable alternative.

SUMMARY

Remember that supplements fall into the three classifications of dietary, sport, and ergogenic. Depending on your sport and overall training goals, there are some supplements that can be of great benefit, while others may not provide as much as food could. Nutrition for athletes is a blend of meeting your health and your performance needs. When you choose a product to enhance your performance, keep in mind that your overall health is of primary importance. Do your homework and read the label and ingredients list on all of the nutritional supplements you currently use or are thinking of using before making a decision to use them or not.

6

Special Considerations for the Athlete

I want to discuss a handful of issues that pertain specifically to your performance as an athlete and that may also be applicable to you in your quest for better health. Some of the issues discussed in this chapter have the potential to impact your performance and health negatively, but, with the right amount of knowledge about each, you can prevent most problems, including the following:

- Dehydration
- Heat cramps
- Hyponatremia
- Immune system depression
- Vegetarianism
- Travel nutrition
- Inflammation
- Iron deficiency anemia

DEHYDRATION

I would bet that you have experienced some degree of dehydration at some point in your training. Why am I so confident about this? Because dehydration is one of the most common ailments among athletes; it doesn't take much to become dehydrated. Forget to eat foods that have a high water content or forget to drink enough fluids throughout the day before your training session, and you will most likely experience some level of dehydration during your workout. Before exploring that topic, let me provide a little background about sweating so that you have an idea of how dehydration can happen so quickly and be such a serious concern.

Sweating is your body's most effective way of cooling itself; when sweat evaporates from your skin, body heat is reduced. Even though sweating is important, if you don't replace the fluids you lose through sweat, it can lead to dehydration and heat illness.

When you are training, the heat that is produced by your muscles exceeds the heat released by your body, and your body temperature rises. The increase in your body temperature causes an increase in sweating and blood flow to your skin. The evaporation of sweat removes heat from your skin. Your body can also lose heat through the processes of radiation, conduction, and convection. In more detail, the four ways that you can lose heat from your body include the following:

1. Radiation: when heat radiates from the body to cooler objects such as buildings, walls, trees, earth, and the air.
2. Conduction: when heat is transferred from the body by direct physical contact with substances at lower temperatures, which happens when you are swimming in cold water.
3. Convection: when heat is transferred by the movement of cool currents of air or water over the body, which can happen when you are training outdoors.
4. Evaporation: when heat is lost when sweat is converted to water vapor, which happens when you are training in a lower-humidity climate.

Your body is made up of approximately 55–65% fluid and has 2–4 million sweat glands. The area that has the most sweat glands is the bottom of the feet; the back is the area that has the fewest. Women have more sweat glands than men, but men have more active sweat glands and typically have a higher sweat rate. When some of the body's fluid is lost through sweat, it affects the cardiovascular system and the ability to control temperature.

How do you know if you are a heavy sweater? After you finish training, notice what I call the "soak factor" of your clothing. If your clothing is dripping wet, you are a heavy sweater. This can also be measured more precisely in a laboratory setting, but the important thing to remember is that if you are a heavy sweater, you may need to stay more on top of your hydration and electrolyte plan during training. More about that later, but let me first explain some of the factors that can influence your sweat rate, so that you can better control them.

- Environment. No matter where you live, chances are good that you train in at least one warm season. The higher temperatures in warmer seasons can cause you to sweat more quickly and to lose more fluids. Add to that the humidity index, and you could be staring dehydration in the eyes. Because humidity affects your body's ability to cool itself, it is harder for sweat to evaporate in hot, humid weather (such as that found in Florida) than in hot, dry weather (such as that found in Colorado in the summer). The dryer the environment, the more likely you can become dehydrated. Get to know your environment and plan your training and hydration needs accordingly. Remember also that even if it is cold, that doesn't mean that you should drink less. Your body is still sweating, and although you may not feel the dryness as much as you would in the heat, you still need to stay hydrated.
- Clothing and equipment. The amount and type of clothing that you wear could contribute to dehydration. By wearing clothing that wicks away sweat and does not hold sweat to your body, you provide an effective medium of sweat dissipation. Wearing 100% cotton, or clothing that does not allow your body heat to be released as efficiently, increases your chances of becoming dehydrated. Sweat suits and rubber suits, commonly worn by weight-class athletes, also increase the

incidence of dehydration. In the case of these athletes, these practices are planned with the goal of dehydrating.

- Fitness and acclimatization. When you increase your fitness level throughout the year, your body becomes more efficient and actually begins to sweat sooner. Some athletes perceive early sweating as a distraction, but this distraction is very beneficial: it is a sign that your body has become better at regulating its core temperature to keep you cool. You may see a significant difference in your sweat rate and amount as you progress throughout your training and competition year.

To understand the true effects of dehydration, look at it from a physiological perspective. The most serious consequence of exercise-induced dehydration is hyperthermia, which places added stress on the cardiovascular system. Because you are already stressing your cardiovascular systems to some extent during training, this added stress is not beneficial. Dehydration causes fluid to be lost throughout the body. As a result, this increases the concentration and osmolality of dissolved substances and particles in your body's fluids, including the concentration of sodium. These increases in osmolality and in sodium concentration reduce blood flow to the skin and thus decrease the rate of sweating.

Another negative consequence of dehydration-induced hyperthermia is a large decline in cardiac output. Cardiac output is the volume of blood pumped by the heart per minute. A decrease in cardiac output can result in less blood—and therefore less oxygen—being delivered to the working muscles, which means that you cannot train as well. This also reduces the transfer of heat from the body core to the skin, so the body core temperature begins to increase. This is extremely hazardous during training and competition.

The primary benefit of sufficient fluid replacement during training is that it helps maintain cardiac output and allows blood flow to the skin to increase to high levels, which promotes heat dissipation from the skin, thereby preventing excessive storage of body heat.

Dehydration can have a negative impact on training and racing with as little as 1% loss of body weight through sweat. If you do the math, you'll realize that this isn't much. If you are a 120-pound athlete, this is only 1.2 pounds. If you are training in a warmer environment, you can easily lose this weight (and probably much more) in a matter of a single training session. Dehydration combined with warmer temperatures could also put you at risk of developing heat illness. Research has shown that dehydration can happen in as little as 30 minutes in a warmer, humid environment.

Avoiding Dehydration

The fluid recommendations change every few years or so in the world of sports nutrition, based on new research. Interestingly, there is a popular scientist and physician in South Africa, Tim Noakes, who has recently challenged the theory of drinking a predetermined amount of fluid at set intervals throughout competition. His point is that it may be okay to compete in a minimally dehydrated state because drinking based on thirst is adequate enough for most athletes. It is an interesting theory, and whether you believe it or not, the take-home message is that it is important to learn when your body is thirsty and to drink accordingly. Drinking ahead of your thirst could actually be detrimental because it might lead to hyponatremia, yet drinking behind your thirst may contribute more to the performance-reducing effects of dehydration. It is definitely a mixed message, but hopefully one that research can help answer in the upcoming years. That said, this method of drinking based on your thirst may not be the best strategy for younger athletes who do not have well-developed thirst mechanisms or for older athletes who have diminished thirst mechanisms.

Heat Cramps

Not only do you have to worry about dehydration, but you also need to be aware of one of the effects of dehydration—heat cramps. Heat cramps can be caused by salt loss and dehydration. They can occur during prolonged training when there has been profuse and repeated sweating. Large losses of fluid and sodium are factors that can predispose you to heat cramps. Because sodium plays an important role in initiating signals from nerves and actions that lead to movement of the muscles, a sodium deficit could short-circuit the coordination of nerves and muscles. This could result in selected motor nerve endings becoming hyperexcitable and result in spontaneous muscle contractions or cramping.

Sweat and Sodium Losses

In warm to hot conditions, it is common to see sweat losses around 1–2 1/2 liters per hour (1 liter is equal to approximately 34 ounces). During longer training sessions or competitions, it is not unheard of for an athlete to lose as much as 10 liters! How much water you lose depends on many factors described previously, including temperature, humidity, solar radiation, intensity of exercise, heat acclimatization status, and your fitness level. An increase in any one of these can increase your sweating.

Sweat is mostly comprised of water, but it also contains many other substances: those most important to this discussion are the minerals sodium, chloride, potassium, calcium, and magnesium. However, the amounts of potassium, calcium, and magnesium are very low compared to the amounts of sodium and chloride.

How much sodium can you lose in a training session or competition? If you are a well-conditioned athlete who is fully acclimatized to the heat, you could have sodium losses of 115–690 milligrams per liter of sweat. If you are not acclimatized to the heat, you can have sodium losses of 920–2,300 milligrams per liter of sweat. And, as your sweat rates go up, so does your loss of sodium. It is common for a heavy sweater to lose 2,500–5,000 milligrams of sodium per hour in a hot environment. Over an extended training session or competition, this could translate into a 15–30% deficit in the total body exchangeable sodium. Note that one teaspoon of salt has 2,400 milligrams of sodium.

Preventing heat cramps begins with replacing fluid and sodium losses during and after training or competition. If you know you are a salty sweater, or if you expect to have a higher sweat rate because of the environment or duration of exercise, you should devise a hydration and electrolyte plan that supports your needs and practice it in training before competitions.

All this talk about hydration and heat cramps wouldn't be complete without explaining the last big hitter among the three heat- and hydration-related issues that endurance athletes face—hyponatremia.

Hyponatremia

Hyponatremia is a disorder in fluid-electrolyte balance that results in an abnormally low plasma sodium concentration. When you combine a hot environment and a salty sweater with a high sweat rate and improper fluid and electrolyte plan, you have a case of hyponatremia just waiting to surface. The sometimes hot and humid environments in which athletes compete can greatly affect performance. This type of environmental stress, combined with the amount you sweat, can spell trouble for you and is certain to result in hyponatremia unless you adopt a sound nutrition plan centered on proper fluid and sodium intake.

Symptoms of Hyponatremia

Some of the symptoms associated with hyponatremia include the following:

- GI discomfort
- Nausea and vomiting
- Throbbing headache
- Restlessness

- Lethargy
- Confusion
- Respiratory distress
- Seizures
- Brainstem herniation
- Death

The risk of developing complications from hyponatremia depends somewhat on the measured level of plasma sodium in your body. The following are the physiological ranges of plasma sodium; these are provided so that you have an idea of the numbers that health professionals refer to:

- Normal: 136–142 mmol/L
- Mild hyponatremia: 125–135 mmol/L
- Severe hyponatremia: <125 mmol/L

Many studies have measured plasma sodium concentrations during and after exercise, and, although the physiological ranges of plasma sodium provides you with an idea of the severity of hyponatremia, the numbers do not always tell the whole story.

For example, athletes have survived hyponatremia when their plasma sodium concentration was in the "severe" category, but others have died under the same conditions. If you think that you may be an at-risk athlete, it is important to account for the following variables in your overall nutrition plan:

- Length of training or competition: longer durations mean a greater chance of developing hyponatremia.
- Sweat rate: heavy sweaters may be more likely to develop hyponatremia if their fluid consumption is not enough to support their sweat losses.
- Sweat sodium content: salty sweaters may be more likely to develop hyponatremia than non-salty sweaters if their sodium intake is not high enough to support their sodium losses.

By knowing these three things ahead of time, you can reduce your risk of developing hyponatremia. Hyponatremia cannot be prevented during training, but the risk can be reduced by proper planning.

Many factors can cause hyponatremia, but the most common is excessive fluid intake. With excessive water intake, there is an increased risk of developing hyponatremia because your body's sodium levels decrease. In addition, sodium loss from sweat is increased, which makes it even easier to dilute your body's sodium content.

Although some researchers believe that hyponatremia is associated with fluid overload, others believe that it is associated with dehydration. What is important to realize is that if you are training or competing in an event in which you have prolonged sweating, this may predispose you to hyponatremia. The balance of fluid intake and sodium intake and the timing of fluid intake become of utmost importance, which is one point of agreement among researchers.

Prevention of Hyponatremia

So now you know what hyponatremia is and the main cause of it, but what you really want to know is how to prevent it. Prevention of hyponatremia must include a combination of knowing if you are an at-risk athlete and knowing how to plan properly to prevent hyponatremia.

Identification of your at-risk status should be your first step. Determine your sweat rate and sweat sodium content. If you want accuracy, the best place to have these measured is in a human performance laboratory that offers this type of testing. If you don't have access to this kind of facility, you can take a more simple but not as quantitative approach. You know during your training whether you have a high sweat rate because, if you do, your clothes are drenched with sweat on a consistent basis by the time you finish a workout (of course, this does depend on the environmental conditions in which you train). Also, if your clothes have a white residue after every training session, you can probably conclude that you are somewhat of a salty sweater. Again, this at-home assessment method does not provide exact numbers, but it helps you determine whether you might be an at-risk athlete.

Once you identify whether you are at risk or not, your next step is to educate and protect yourself. If you are at risk, adopt the following strategies in your nutrition plan:

- Consume sodium with adequate fluids during exercise. Interdepartmental fluid shifts (when the sodium concentration inside your body increases or decreases because of more or less water intake) can happen when too much sodium is introduced into the body without adequate fluid. Hypernatremia can develop as a result of harboring too much sodium without enough fluid. Then you have a whole other issue to worry about!
- Avoid overdrinking. I cannot emphasize this point more strongly. Stick to your fluid and sodium intake plan that you determine beforehand and do not drink ahead of your thirst.
- Limit prehydration to only water. Failure to do this can lower your blood sodium before the event begins and leave you behind in your sodium intake plan.

Knowing the risks and symptoms of hyponatremia is important any time of the year that you are training. Knowing your individual sweat rate and sweat sodium concentration is helpful so that you can plan your fluid and sodium needs. However, if you can't have these measured, simply follow the fluid and sodium guidelines presented earlier in this book and fine-tune them to your body as you find necessary.

IMMUNE SYSTEM DEPRESSION

Regular, moderate exercise is beneficial for maintaining good health, but more intense workouts can suppress the immune system and increase your chances of getting sick. The increased susceptibility for illness after exercise is thought to be related to the increase in stress hormones during and after exercise. This can last between 3 and 72 hours, and, during this time, viruses and bacteria can exert their negative effects on your body.

Cortisol

Cortisol, one of the main culprits in the stress hormone family, is a hormone controlled by the adrenal cortex (your body's factory for producing steroid hormones) and is known to be the regulator of the immune system. Its primary functions are to increase protein breakdown in your muscles, inhibit the uptake of glucose into your body's cells, and increase the breakdown of fats. Cortisol levels can have a negative impact on many different areas in your body, including sleep, mood, bone health, ligament health, cardiovascular health, and athletic performance.

What does this all of this mean for athletes? High levels of cortisol may result when you don't pay close attention to your daily nutrition. A chronically elevated amount of cortisol causes fat, protein, and carbohydrates to be mobilized quickly; while this is happening, two other hormones, testosterone and dehydroepiaandrosterone (DHEA), decrease. Your body then enters a constant state of muscle breakdown and suppressed immune function. It's a vicious cycle that repeats itself over and over when you don't follow a sound eating program.

In addition, high cortisol levels can put you at greater risk for developing upper respiratory tract infections (often referred to as URTIs). Some researchers have shown that using the ratio of anabolic to catabolic steroids (i.e., the ratio of testosterone to cortisol) can provide results that can help assess an athlete's training state. A ratio that favors increased cortisol can indicate overtraining.

If you train in a carbohydrate-depleted state (i.e., follow a daily low-carbohydrate diet), you could experience a greater amount of cortisol in your body. Unfortunately, high-intensity and long-duration training both increase cortisol levels. If you are trying to improve your speed or explosive power or are training for an event lasting longer than 3–4 hours, chances are that you have a high amount of cortisol in your body. This remains elevated for about two hours after you finish training, which means, as I keep saying, that your daily nutrition plan is of utmost importance.

But how do you actually know if your cortisol levels are high? It just so happens that a few easy-to-recognize symptoms can lead you to the answer without having your cortisol levels measured. Symptoms of high cortisol levels include mood swings, lack of motivation to train, and loss of muscle and appetite.

I keep mentioning the power of nutrition to help control cortisol levels. Regulating and controlling cortisol levels begins during the daily nutrition that leads up to your training sessions. Carbohydrates can help decrease the cortisol response, so if you follow a daily eating program that has enough carbohydrates to support your energy needs, you are taking the first step in cortisol control. Going into a hard workout without adequate carbohydrate stores sets you up for improper recovery, as well as for the negative impact of high cortisol levels following exercise. Some good research has also demonstrated that the addition of glutamine and BCAA during your post exercise nutrition plan can also help modulate cortisol release.

VEGETARIANISM

The term "vegetarianism" is used loosely with many athletes—from those who do not eat red meat to those who do not eat any animal products at all. I encounter many athletes who claim to be vegetarian when, in fact, they are not because they may not fully understand the different classifications associated with vegetarianism. Here are some of the more common categories of vegetarian diets:

- Lacto-vegetarian: no animal foods except for milk and milk products (yogurt, cheese, cottage cheese).

- Lacto-ovo-vegetarian: no animal foods except for eggs, milk, and milk products.
- Vegan: no animal foods at all.

I have met some athletes who fall into a couple of the different categories and those who also eat fish but no other meats. It doesn't really matter what type of vegetarianism is followed or whether it is for ethical, moral, or health purposes. What is important is how this can affect your health and performance.

Effects of Vegetarianism

When you are fueling up for your training session or competition, remember that you want to choose foods that enhance your health and improve your performance. Optimal performance can only come with good health. Athletes who follow any type of vegetarian diet seem to have a lower risk of developing diseases such as diabetes and heart disease in later years of life. Unfortunately, much of the scientific research is focused on health effects of vegetarianism and not specifically on performance.

Of course, there are some challenges when it comes to following a vegetarian eating plan. Protein food sources are present, but it takes a bit more work to include them into your daily nutrition plan based on what type of vegetarianism you follow. It is easy to find a piece of chicken or glass of milk, but when you choose not to eat those food items, the hunt for protein is more challenging. Here is a list of non-meat options that can help you maintain a good balance between protein and carbohydrate:

- Soy milk
- Tofu
- Edamame
- Quinoa (a grain that is a good source of protein)
- Walnuts, almonds
- Kidney and black beans
- Tempeh

- Hummus
- Peanut, soynut, or almond butter

For many athletes thinking of adopting a vegetarian lifestyle, it can be easier to progress from minimizing animal product consumption to avoiding it altogether over time. I personally believe in following this natural progression for most athletes because it is easier to learn about substitute foods and maintain being a vegetarian. Keep in mind the following dietary concerns if you decide to move away from an animal-based to a plant-based diet:

1. Total energy: most vegetarian diets are high in carbohydrate-rich foods, such as fruits, vegetables, and grains, that have ample fiber and are very filling. This could result in not eating enough calories to support training and competition. I have worked with many vegan athletes who had problems maintaining their weight. Good strategies to include more calories in your eating program are to eat nuts, peanut butter, soy products, and meat substitutes.

2. Protein: vegetarian athletes who do not eat any type of meat or dairy foods could have low protein intakes. During some times of the training year, protein intake should be higher to support physical needs. Higher nonmeat protein-foods include nuts, tofu, soy milk, and some whole-grain-based cereals.

3. Iron: vegetarian athletes are at greater risk for having low iron stores because the most absorbable type of iron (heme iron) is only found in animal products. Nonheme iron, found in plant sources, contains iron, but it is in lower amounts and is not as absorbable. Iron is needed to help the muscles get oxygen; low amounts of iron could cause fatigue and poor performance. Female athletes are more affected than males because of the monthly blood loss from menstruation. Be sure to include good non-animal sources of iron, including spinach, broccoli, almonds, oatmeal, and iron-fortified cereals. Consuming a source of vitamin C, such as drinking

orange juice, with these types of foods can help the body absorb more iron.

4. Calcium: for those vegetarian athletes who do not drink milk or any dairy foods, calcium intake may be low. Calcium is very important for healthy bones and also muscle contractions. Alternate sources of calcium-rich foods include fortified cereals, tofu, soy milk, and green leafy vegetables.

5. Vitamin B12: there is no active form of this vitamin in any plant foods, and, because vitamin B12 is involved in the breakdown of foods to energy, low amounts can be detrimental for performance. Pure vegan athletes are at risk of developing anemia from deficiency of this vitamin, and this can lead to fatigue. Fortified foods are the top choice and include cereals and soy products.

It is very possible to follow any type of vegetarian eating program and still be healthy and perform well. The tricks are to become more educated about plant-based food options and to choose many varieties and options of fruits, vegetables, nuts, legumes, soy products, and meat alternatives. I'll be honest—it takes some planning in the initial stages of adopting a vegetarian lifestyle, but it becomes much easier once you broaden your knowledge of food.

TRAVEL NUTRITION

Competition season brings more travel to an athlete's already busy schedule. Whether you are traveling across the United States or internationally, jet lag can pose a performance problem. Timing of your sleep/wake cycle is regulated by a biological clock located in your brain. When you rapidly cross time zones, this clock cannot adjust quickly enough, which causes biological processes to become disrupted and "out of whack."

The severity of jet lag is variable and is dependent upon the number of time zones crossed, the direction traveled (east or west), and athlete susceptibility. Jet lag does not occur if you stay in the same time zone, because there is not a change to your biological clock. However, within the same time zone, typical responses to travel can occur, which include stress, dehydration, and muscle stiffness, so it is important to be aware of these even when you are traveling a short distance to a competition within the same time zone.

Jet lag not only makes you feel groggy and tired, but, more important, it can have a negative impact on your performance because of the following associated consequences:

- Decreased alertness
- Decreased concentration
- Reductions in anaerobic power
- Prolonged reaction time
- Reduced strength

Typically, the rule of thumb states that it takes about one day for your biological clock to adjust to each time zone you cross. However, it is possible to shorten this time by following these specific nutrition guidelines as you travel to and from your competition.

Two weeks prior to travel
- If you are flying, contact the airline you will be flying with and arrange for a special in-flight meal to include a low-fat, vegetarian, or fruit option.
- If you are driving, be sure to locate safe and familiar eating establishments along the way so that you can have planned meals that you are normally used to eating. Also identify rest stop locations for bathroom use.

Six days to one day prior to travel
- Shop for your favorite "safe foods" that you can eat in case the food presented to you is not to your liking. Have at least 4–5 staple foods that are "GI safe," that is, do not cause discomfort in your digestive system.

Two days to one day prior to travel

- Pack your personal travel nutrition kit. Remember to pack enough for the flight (or car ride), layovers, wait times, and delays. Include the following:
  - Water bottles
  - Sandwiches or portable meals
  - Fruits (fresh, dried)
  - Fruit juice
  - Energy bars, crackers, dry cereal, trail mix, bagels
  - Powdered sports drink and protein powders
  - Extra sandwich bags

- Remain hydrated. Be sure that your urine is clear to pale-yellow in color throughout each of these days.

On the day of travel

  - Ensure that you are well hydrated.
  - Put your travel nutrition kit in your carry-on luggage or in a bag close to where you are sitting in the car. Having your nutrition within close proximity is crucial.

In flight or in a car

  - Immediately adjust your eating schedule to your destination time zone (not to the airline's food serving schedule if you are flying).
  - Consume a minimum of 8 ounces of fluid every hour.
  - Monitor your hydration status by the frequency of using the bathroom. Try to urinate every 2–3 hours.
  - Avoid alcohol.
  - If you consume caffeine, do it in the destination time zone and in low amounts.

These nutrition recommendations help lessen the effects of jet lag, but remember that many other variables are involved with jet lag. Nutrition is but one piece of the puzzle.

As with any type of travel preparation, be sure to give your nutrition preparation just as much attention as you do packing for competition.

INFLAMMATION

Aerobic capacity is reduced when the body is in an inflammatory state. This raises obvious concerns for any athlete because systemic inflammation can have a negative effect on both health and performance.

The basic concept of this detriment to performance is linked to the lining of the artery, often referred to as the endothelial lining. When this lining becomes inflamed, there is greater vasoconstriction and less blood delivered to working muscles. This translates into less oxygen and nutrient delivery and less waste removal from the muscles. In addition to blood flow mechanics, there has also been some association between pulmonary inflammation and asthma, which can significantly affect oxygen uptake in athletes who have problems with asthma.

Basics of Inflammation

Invaders to the body, such as bacteria and viruses, are encountered quite often throughout the day, but they are normally attacked and destroyed by the body's internal inflammatory processes. A small amount of inflammation is needed, but adding strenuous exercise can increase the inflammatory response beyond the body's regulatory controls.

There are two main types of inflammation: classic and silent. Classic is most common because it is the type that can be seen by obvious bruising and is felt with pain. This type of inflammation is usually remedied by rest, ice, compression, and elevation, and the body is very good at responding and initiating the recovery process.

Silent inflammation, on the other hand, can have significant negative health and performance effects. This type of inflammation is often involved in disease states such as heart disease, Alzheimer's, rheumatoid arthritis, and cancer. There is no visual swelling or bruising. In fact, the only way to find out the amount of inflammation in the body is through a blood test that looks at the level of C-reactive protein (CRP). CRP is a marker of total body inflammation, which can begin at a very young age. This type of inflammation is more difficult to manage, mostly because of its asymptomatic condition.

The Science of Inflammation

It is common knowledge these days which foods should and should not be used to improve performance or speed recovery, but, as of late, more attention has been brought to fats. Once touted as "bad," certain fats can actually improve the body's ability to combat inflammation and improve exercise performance. The metabolism and effects of fatty acids are quite complex, and it is important to understand on a basic level that different types of fats can either increase or decrease inflammation by "turning on and off" certain hormones.

The types of fat that are highly related to inflammation include saturated, trans, and the polyunsaturates omega-3 and omega-6. Saturated and trans fats promote inflammation and should be reduced. The polyunsaturates have a different effect on the body and are more important to understand regarding the inflammatory response.

Omega-6 fats, found in safflower, soybean, corn, and sunflower oils, are broken down into two main constituents: arachidonic acid (AA) and gamma-linolenic acid (GLA). Too much AA leads to inflammation. Because the typical U.S. diet is overloaded with vegetable oils, AA is produced in copious amounts, in fact, 20–30 times more than is needed. GLA, although it is also an omega-6 fat, has anti-inflammatory properties, because it is not converted to the pro-inflammatory AA. GLA is converted to diho-mogamma-linolenic acid (DGLA), which competes with AA in the breakdown; if it wins, it negates the pro-inflammatory effects of AA. Consuming too much omega-6 fat can lead to a greater amount of inflammation in the body as a result of high levels of AA.

Eating the omega-3 polyunsaturated fats leads to very positive health outcomes. In addition to helping control inflammation, omega-3 fats have been proven to do the following:

- Decrease risk for coronary artery disease
- Decrease hypertension
- Improve insulin sensitivity
- Reduce tenderness in joints for individuals with rheumatoid arthritis
- Protect against stroke caused by plaque buildup and blood clots
- Lower triglycerides and raise levels of high-density lipoproteins (HDL, the healthy cholesterol)

Omega-3 fats are converted to the beneficial compounds that most individuals have heard of: eicosapentaenoic acid (EPA) and docosahexanoic acid (DHA). The same enzyme is shared in converting omega-3 fats in food products to EPA and DHA as is used in the conversion of omega-6 fats to AA. Because of the high amount of vegetable oil and processed foods, laden with omega-6 fats and less omega-3 fats that is eaten by some individuals, the conversion to the pro-inflammatory AA happens more often.

Inflammation and Food

Part of the understanding of the interaction of food and inflammation begins with what most athletes already know: too much low-density lipoprotein (LDL) cholesterol can negatively affect health. Too much of this cholesterol can cause the cascade of inflammatory events; the oxidation of LDL is of particular concern in this inflammatory process. Therefore, it makes sense to control this as much as possible by reducing LDL cholesterol through choosing the correct foods that are particularly low in saturated fat.

As mentioned previously, certain fats increase or decrease inflammation. There are a host of other foods that also contribute, either positively or negatively, to the inflammation process. In no specific order, a brief list of foods that can produce a pro-inflammatory response include the following:

- Refined starches and sugars (white bread, cereals, candy, soft drinks, pastries)
- Sweets (cakes, cookies, pies)
- Fried foods (high in saturated and trans fats)
- Processed meats (sausage, pepperoni, lunch meats)

In contrast, the following include top food choices that have anti-inflammatory properties:

- Extra virgin olive oil
- Turmeric spice
- Pineapple
- Fresh fruits (especially berries)
- Fresh vegetables (spinach, broccoli, carrots)
- Pumpkin seeds
- Wild salmon
- Flax products (ground flax is preferred over whole flax seeds)
- Grass-fed game meat (bison, venison)
- Whole grains
- Almonds
- Green tea

When it comes to inflammation and foods, the information can be a bit confusing and contradictory from time to time. Luckily, a rating system has been developed and makes choosing anti-inflammatory foods easier. This system is called the Inflammation Factor Rating™ system; it provides an inflammation rating number to foods. Although there is not a scale with good and bad ranges, this system provides, at minimum, enough information for athletes to choose pro- or anti-inflammatory foods. This rating system uses information such as content of sugar, vitamin and mineral, and saturated and healthier fats to determine the inflammation rating. Processed foods and those with high sugar, saturated fat, and trans fat content top the pro-inflammatory list; foods rich in lean protein, vitamins, minerals, healthy fats, and nonrefined or processed carbohydrates top the anti-inflammatory list.

Some of the higher inflammatory foods according to this rating scale include the following:

- Plain bagel
- Corn flakes
- Chocolate ice cream
- Farm-raised Atlantic salmon

In contrast, the following foods have a lower inflammation factor:

- Wild Atlantic salmon
- Carrots
- Broccoli
- Olive oil
- Raw spinach

It is important to remember that just because a food has a high inflammation factor rating, it does not mean that you should not include it in your nutrition plan. Combining foods and producing an overall anti-inflammatory score are the important keys to success in meal preparation.

This rating system does not provide an extensive list by any means, but there is an online resource that offers information about the inflammation factor of foods. The Nutrition Data Web site has begun to adopt the Inflammation Factor Rating™ system to make it easier to choose foods based on their inflammation score.

Too much inflammation has a negative effect on health and performance. If left unchanged, chronic inflammation can have a significant impact on health and exercise performance; by simple alterations of the type and amount of fat in your nutrition plan, inflammation can be controlled.

IRON DEFICIENCY ANEMIA

Iron is one of the most common supplements that some athletes take. Unfortunately, this particular mineral is often misunderstood. I have experienced many situations where athletes take iron supplements without clinical justification; this is unsafe. One of the most detrimental things an athlete can do is take an iron supplement without first having a blood test for full iron stores that can identify a deficiency.

About Iron

The body has approximately 3.5–4.5 grams of iron storage. About two-thirds of this is found in hemoglobin, and the rest is distributed in the liver, spleen, and bone marrow, with small amounts in myoglobin. Even though not all athletes require supplemental iron, increased risk of iron deficiency is often identified by the following symptoms:

- Unrecognized bleeding from the intestinal tract
- Hematuria (presence of blood in the urine)
- Heavy sweating (iron is found in small amounts in sweat)
- Foot strike hemolysis (destruction of red blood cells by the impact of the foot strike on the ground)
- Females who regularly menstruate
- Inflammation (can lead to an increase in hepcidin-a protein, which reduces gastrointestinal iron absorption)
- Restriction of calories

Athletes who experience one or more of these symptoms are encouraged to obtain a full iron stores blood work analysis through their physician. This is the first step in the process.

Iron plays many roles in the body, some of which include the following:

- Mitochondrial oxidative enzymes
- Thyroid hormone metabolism
- Neural function
- Immune function
- Erythropoiesis (formation of new red blood cells)

One of the most important roles iron plays is as a component of the protein hemoglobin, which carries oxygen from the lungs to the body's cells. Because one red blood cell contains about 250 million hemoglobin molecules, a higher level of iron can mean higher aerobic capacity and better performance.

Iron stores can be difficult to maintain for athletes because iron absorption from a typical Western diet ranges from 10–35%; following a vegetarian diet results in much less iron absorption, from 1–20%. It is important to remember this when choosing foods. Some foods are higher in iron, but keep in mind that the absorption rates may still be low, comparatively speaking. To add to this challenge, iron inhibitors can decrease iron absorption even more. These include calcium, zinc (although maybe not when consumed as food rather than as a supplement), phytates and fiber found in whole grains and nuts, tannins found in coffee and tea, and bran and soy products. Additionally, athletes with Celiac disease or Crohn's disease may also have lower rates of iron absorption because of the affects on the GI system. In contrast, there are iron promoters that have or promote a higher rate of absorption. These include meat, fish, poultry, broccoli, brussels sprouts, tomatoes, potatoes, green and red peppers, and other foods rich in vitamin C.

The two types of iron in foods are heme and non-heme. Heme iron comes from animal sources, such as beef, chicken, shrimp, oysters, sardines, and fish; it has a high absorption rate. Non-heme iron comes from vegetable sources, such as enriched cereals, blackstrap molasses, pumpkin seeds, beans, lentils, and tofu; it has a much lower absorption rate versus heme iron sources.

Signs and Symptoms of Low Iron Stores

The most common symptom associated with iron deficiency anemia is fatigue that worsens with exertion during exercise. Fatigue is common in sport and can have many different causes, such as other nutritional imbalances, illness, or stress. If an athlete experiences normal fatigue throughout the day and the fatigue is not worsened with exercise, the cause is likely not iron deficiency by itself; however, a blood test should be done to rule out iron problems. The following are also possible symptoms of iron deficiency anemia:

- Decreased performance
- Sleepiness and fatigue (outside of normal)
- Poor concentration
- Moodiness or irritability
- Always feeling cold
- Decreased immune function
- Eating non-nutritive substances, such as dirt, clay, or ice (often referred to as pica)

A full blood iron laboratory panel is the best way to assess iron status. A number of clinical markers are used to explain iron status; the following is a brief description of these markers.

- Hematocrit: proportion of blood volume that consists of red blood cells
- Hemoglobin: iron-containing oxygen-transport protein in red blood cells
- Mean corpuscular volume: a measure of the average volume of a red blood cell
- Ferritin: a globular protein complex that is the main intracellular iron storage protein
- Serum iron: the level of iron in the liquid portion of blood
- Transferrin: a plasma protein in the blood that binds to iron and transports it

- Total iron-binding capacity: a measure of the total amount of iron that transferrin can bind
- Transferrin saturation: the percentage of iron-binding sites occupied by iron on transferrin
- Soluble transferrin receptor: a trans-membrane glycoprotein that controls the uptake of circulating iron into cells

Serum ferritin, one of the most common clinical markers used in the assessment of iron deficiency, is not tapped into until levels of iron become too low to support demands. For example, if the body is using and excreting more iron than it is receiving from food, the ferritin level slowly declines. If an iron deficiency is suspected, an athlete should visit a sports physician and receive a complete blood count (CBC) and full iron panel. It is important to choose a health professional (physician, sport dietitian, physiologist) who has experience with iron deficiency because normal lab values, often seen on most blood work reports, may not represent an athlete's normal state.

It is also important to keep in mind that being dehydrated before testing can cause higher values for some of these iron markers. Be sure to be well hydrated and in a somewhat rested state (not the day or two after a hard or long run) because this also affects iron blood markers.

Iron Deficiency Stages

There are three stages of iron deficiency, all with different blood marker fluctuations, which is yet another reason why athletes should receive iron stores blood testing on a frequent basis. Stage one is iron depletion, the most mild form of iron deficiency. Normally, serum ferritin levels are decreased, and if detected early enough, this stage can be easily managed through food; in most cases, it does not require supplementation. Stage two is iron deficiency without anemia, which is characterized by a low serum ferritin, a decrease in the percentage of transferrin saturation, and an increase in total iron-binding capacity. This also can be treated with food if it is caught early enough; supplementation may be needed. Stage three, anemia, is the most serious of the stages and includes all of the previously mentioned blood clinical markers in addition to a decrease in hemoglobin. There are various types of anemia; identifying the type may facilitate the treatment protocol.

- Macrocytic: red blood cells are larger than normal; the most common is called megaloblastic or pernicious anemia. It is caused be a deficiency of vitamin B_{12} or folic acid.
- Microcytic: red blood cells are smaller than normal; the main cause is iron deficiency anemia.
- Normocytic: red blood cells are normal size but low in quantity, with a low hemoglobin level. Typical causes are chronic illness, medications, pregnancy, and hemolysis.

- Sports: this is not a clinically recognized type but is common among athletes in the initial phases of training. Because of a higher plasma volume (training response), iron in the body appears to be diluted, and hemoglobin levels are lower. An athlete should not worry or supplement with iron if this is seen; the body adapts. Performance has not been shown to be compromised.

Improving Iron Stores

Training

Based on the particular laboratory and the geographical region, normal ranges for iron markers differ, so it is important to receive a baseline test in the normal living environment, not during a short-term visit to another location. Ideally, have this done during the off-season cycle (lower training load) because of the linear relationship that typically exists between iron stores and training status.

Generally speaking, high-volume training can cause a decrease in iron stores; therefore, it is important to account for this by periodizing an athlete's nutrition, specifically iron in this case, based on training load changes. I recommend a 6-week iron focus for athletes leading up to a higher training load or if they are traveling to a high altitude. This amount of time allows the body to increase its iron stores to prevent a significant performance-decreasing effect during the training cycle. I note that this strategy is underutilized.

Food

As previously stated, training increases the demand placed on the body's iron stores. But, depending on the athlete and on current iron stores, it is possible to improve iron stores through a well-structured eating program. Non vegetarians should specifically pay attention to consuming more foods containing heme iron; vegetarians have a greater challenge because foods containing non-heme iron constitute the majority of their iron intake. Athletes who are vegetarian must make a concerted effort to choose enriched foods and eat non-heme sources of iron at each meal. The following charts represent the Recommended Dietary Allowance and Tolerable Upper Intakes of iron as references.

Table 6.1
Recommended Dietary Allowances for Iron

Age	Males mg/day	Females mg/day	Pregnancy mg/day	Lactation mg/day
9–13 years	8	8	n/a	n/a
14–18 years	11	15	27	10
19–50 years	8	18	27	9
51+ years	8	8	n/a	n/a

Table 6.2
Tolerable Upper Intakes for Iron

Age	Males mg/day	Females mg/day	Pregnancy mg/day	Lactation mg/day
9–13 years	40	40	n/a	n/a
14–18 years	45	45	45	45
19+ years	45	45	45	45

Supplementation

In a perfect world, supplementation would not be necessary, but, for some athletes, it may be a necessity in addition to a sound, iron-rich nutrition program. For those with clinically diagnosed iron deficiency anemia, it is important to focus on eating foods that are high in iron along with taking an iron supplement. If iron stores are too low, it is extremely difficult to increase these through food alone, especially if an athlete is in a high training load or race season.

Iron supplements can be misused; thus I highly recommend that you consult with a sports physician or a sports dietitian before taking any supplement. There could be complications of iron overload, namely the development of hemochromatosis (caused by a genetic defect that affects the ability to regulate and absorb the iron in the body).

Taking iron supplements does not fall into the "more must be better" category; they can have very dangerous side effects. In fact, iron becomes less absorbable when taken in higher quantities. Additionally, supplemental iron may cause certain GI distress, such as constipation. I often see this when athletes take supplements containing ferrous sulfate, gluconate, or fumarate. Although there are many types of iron supplements on the market, there is a type of iron that is more absorbable (up to 75% compared with the others previously mentioned with absorption rates around 10%) and thus lower quantities are required: it is called ferrous bisglycinate, with the trade name "ferrochel" and is found in stand-alone form and in multi-vitamins. The additional benefit is that it has very few to no negative GI side effects and does not affect other mineral absorption.

Replenishment of iron stores typically takes about 6–8 weeks, depending on the stage, and, in cases of the first stage of iron deficiency, supplementation may not be necessary. Athletes should emphasize eating iron-rich foods, pay special attention to when training load changes are scheduled, and be sure to have frequent blood tests performed to monitor the status of iron stores throughout the year in relation to training, competitions, and possible supplementation. Iron supplements should be used wisely and only after clinical iron stores blood testing has been completed and evaluated by a qualified sports physician or sports dietitian.

SUMMARY

Not every athlete has experience with all of the special topics mentioned in this chapter. But it is important is to understand the basic concepts, causes, and symptoms so that you can manage your body and, hopefully, prevent many of these conditions from taking hold. However, if you do experience some of these, having knowledge about what to do becomes paramount. Being proactive instead of reactive may just save your competition season.

Bibliography

Acheton, J, Gleeson, M and Jeukendrup, AE. Determination of the exercise intensity that elicits maximal fat oxidation. Med Sci Sports Exerc 34: 92–97. 2002.

ACSM Position Statement. Nutrition and Athletic Performance. Med Sci Sports Exer 41(3): 709–731. 2009.

ADA Position Statement. Vegetarian Diets. J Am Diet Assoc 109: 1266–1282. 2009.

Aguilo, A, et al. Antioxidant diet supplementation enhances aerobic performance in amateur sportsmen. J Sports Sci 25(11): 1203–1210. 2007.

Antonio, J and Street, C. Glutamine: A potentially useful supplement for athletes. Can J Appl Physiol 24: 1–14. 1999.

Astorino, TA and Roberson, DW. Efficacy of acute caffeine ingestion for short-term high-intensity exercise performance: A systematic review. J Strength Cond Res 24(1): 257–265. 2010.

Avois, L, Robinson, N, Saudan, C, Baume, N, Mangin, P and Saugy, M. Central nervous system stimulants and sport practice. Br J Sports Med 40 (Suppl 1): 16–20. 2006.

Barham, JB, et al. Addition of eicosapentaenoic acid to gamma-linolenic acid supplemented diets prevents serum arachidonic acid accumulation in humans. J Nutr 130: 1925–1931. 2000.

Bassit, RA, et al. Branched-chain amino acid supplementation and the immune response of long-distance athletes. Nutrition 18(5): 376–379. 2002.

Bassit, RA, Sawada, LA, Bacarau, RFP, Navarro, F and Costa Rosa, LFBP. The effect of BCAA supplementation upon the immune response of triathletes. Med Sci Sports Exerc 32: 1214–1219. 2000.

Beard, J, Tobin, B. Iron status and exercise. Am J Clin Nutr 72 (2 Suppl): 594S–597S. 2000.

Birnbaum, LJ and Herbst, JD. Physiologic effects of caffeine on cross-country runners. J Strength Cond Res 18(3): 463–465. 2004.

Bompa, TO. *Periodization training for sports.* Champaign, IL: Human Kinetics. 1999.

Braun, B, Grediagin, A, Mazzeo, RS, Cymerman, A and Friedlander, AL. Cytokine responses at high altitude: Effects of exercise and antioxidants at 4300 m. Med Sci Sports Exerc 38(2): 276–285. 2006.

Brooks, GA and Mercier, J. Balance of carbohydrate and lipid utilization during exercise: The "crossover" concept. J Appl Physiol 76: 2253–2261. 1994.

Brooks, GA and Trimmer, JK. Glucose kinetics during high-intensity exercise and the crossover concept. J Appl Physiol 80: 1073–1075. 1996.

Bucci, LR. Selected herbals and human exercise performance. Am J Clin Nutr 72(2): 624–636. 2000.

Burke, LM. Caffeine and sports performance. Appl Physiol Nutr Metab 33(6): 1319–1334. 2008.

Burke, LM, et al. Effect of coingestion of fat and protein with carbohydrate feedings on muscle glycogen storage. J Appl Physiol 78: 2187–2192. 1995.

Burke, LM, Cox, GR, Culmmings, NK and Desbrow, B. Guidelines for daily carbohydrate intake: Do athletes achieve them? Sports Med 31: 267–299. 2001.

Burke, LM and Reed, RSD. Diet patterns of elite Australian male triathletes. Phys Sports Med 15: 140–155. 1987.

Bussau, VA, Fairchild, TJ, Rao, A, Steele, P and Fournier, PA. Carbohydrate loading in human muscle: An improved 1-day protocol. Eur J Appl Physiol 87(3): 290–295. 2002.

Butterfield, G. Amino acids and high protein diets. In: Lamb D, Williams, M, eds. *Perspectives in exercise science and sports medicine.* Carmel, IN: Cooper Publishing Group; 1991; 87–122.

Carbohydrates and exercise. In: Dunford, M, ed. *Sports nutrition. A guide for the professional working with active people.* Sports, Cardiovascular, and Wellness Nutritionist Practice Group, The American Dietetic Association; 2000; 14–33.

Castell, L. Glutamine supplementation in vitro and in vivo, in exercise and in immunodepression. Sports Med 33(5): 323–345. 2003.

Childs, A, et al. Supplementation with vitamin C and N-acetylcysteine increases oxidative stress in humans after an acute muscle injury induced by eccentric exercise. Free Radic Biol Med 31(6): 745–753. 2001.

Close, GL, Ashton, T, Cable, T, Doran, D, Holloway, C, McArdle, F and MacLaren, DP. Ascorbic acid supplementation does not attenuate post-exercise muscle soreness following muscle-damaging exercise but may delay the recovery process. Br J Nutr 95(5): 976–981. 2006.

Compher, C, Frankenfield, D, Keim, N and Roth-Yousey, L. Best practice methods to apply to measurement of resting metabolic rate in adults: a systematic review. J Am Diet Assoc 106(6): 881–903. 2006.

Coombes, JS and McNaughton, LR. Effects of branched-chain amino acid supplementation on serum creatine kinase and lactate dehydrogenase after prolonged exercise. J Sports Med Phys Fitness 40: 240–246. 2000.

Cortes, B, et al. Acute effects of high-fat meals enriched with walnuts or olive oil on postprandial endothelial function. J Amer Coll Cardiol 48(8): 1666–1671. 2006.

Costill, DL, Dalsky, GP and Fink, WJ. Effects of caffeine ingestion on metabolism and exercise performance. Med Sci Sports Exercise 10: 155–158. 1978.

Cox, GR, et al. Effect of different protocols of caffeine intake on metabolism and endurance performance. J Appl Physiol 93(3): 990–999. 2002.

Davison, G and Gleeson, M. Influence of acute vitamin C and/or carbohydrate ingestion on hormonal, cytokine, and immune responses to prolonged exercise. Int J Sport Nutr Exerc Metab 15(5): 465–479. 2005.

Davison, GW, Hughes, CM and Bell RA. Exercise and mononuclear cell DNA damage: The effects of antioxidant supplementation. Int J Sport Nutr Exerc Metab 15(5): 480–492. 2005.

Dietary reference intakes for calcium, phosphorus, magnesium, vitamin D and fluoride, 1997. National Academies Press. Accessible at http://www.nap.edu.

Dietary reference intakes for thiamin, riboflavin, niacin, vitamin B_6, folate, vitamin B_{12}, pantothenic acid, biotin and choline, 1998. National Academies Press. Accessible at http://www.nap.edu.

Dietary reference intakes for vitamin C, vitamin E, selenium and carotenoids, 2000. National Academies Press. Accessible at http://www.nap.edu.

Dietary reference intakes for vitamin A, vitamin K, arsenic, boron, chromium, copper, iodine, iron, manganese, molybdenum, nickel, silicon, vanadium and zinc, 2001. National Academies Press. Accessible at http://www.nap.edu.

Doherty, M, Smith, P, Hughes, M and Davison, R. Caffeine lowers perceptual response and increases power output during high-intensity cycling. J Sports Sci 22(7): 637–643. 2004.

Dohm GL, et al. Metabolic response to exercise after fasting. J Appl Physiol 61: 1363–1368. 1986.

Eden, BD and Abernathy, PJ. Nutritional intake during an ultraendurance running race. Int J Sport Nutr 4: 166–174. 1994.

Essig, D, Costill, DL and Van Handel, RJ. Effects of caffeine ingestion on utilization of muscle glycogen and lipid during leg ergometer cycling. Int J Sports Med 1: 86–89. 1980.

Evans, WJ. Vitamin E, vitamin C, and exercise. Am J Clin Nutr 72(2 Suppl): 647S–652S. 2000.

Fallon, KE. Utility of hematological and iron-related screening in elite athletes. Clin J Sport Med 14(3): 145–152. 2004.

Finaud, J, Lae, G and Filaire, E. Oxidative stress relationship with exercise and training. Sports Med 36(4): 327–358. 2006.

Fisher, SM, et al. Influence of caffeine on exercise performance in habitual caffeine users. Int J Sports Med 7: 276–280. 1986.

Friedlander, AL, Casazza, GA, Horning, MA, Buddinger, TF and Brooks, GA. Effects of exercise intensity and training on lipid metabolism in young women. Am J Physiol 275: E853–863. 1998.

Friedlander, AL, Jacobs, KA, Fattor, JA, Horning, MA, Hagobian, TA, Bauer, TA, Wolfel, EE and Brooks, GA. Contributions of working muscle to whole body lipid metabolism vary with exercise intensity and training. Am J Physiol Endocrinol Metab 292: E107–E116. 2007.

Gabel, KA, Aldous, A. and Edgington, C. Dietary intake of two elite male cyclists during a 10-day, 2,050-mile ride. Int J Sport Nutr 5: 56–61. 1995.

Ganio, MS, Klau, JF, Casa, DJ, Armstrong, LE and Maresh, CM. Effect of caffeine on sport-specific endurance performance: A systematic review. J Strength Cond Res 23(1): 315–324. 2009.

Garcia-Roves, PM, Terrados, N, Fernandez, SF and Patterson, AM. Macronutrient intakes of top-level cyclists during continuous competition-change in feeding pattern. Int J Sport Med 19: 61–67. 1998.

Gleeson, M, Nieman, D and Pedersen, B. Exercise, nutrition, and immune function. J Sport Sci 22: 115–125. 2004.

Halson, SL, et al. Immunological responses to overreaching in cyclists. Med Sci Sports Exerc 35(5): 854–861. 2003.

Hill, CA, et al. Influence of beta-alanine supplementation on skeletal muscle carnosine concentrations and high intensity cycling capacity. Amino Acids 32(2): 225–233. 2007.

Hill, CA, Harris, RC, Kim, HJ, Harris, BD, Sale, C, Boobis, LH, Kim, CK and Wise, JA. Influence of beta-alanine supplementation on skeletal muscle carnosine concentrations and high intensity cycling capacity. Amino Acids 32(2): 225–233. 2007.

Hiscock, N, et al. Glutamine supplementation further enhances exercise-induced plasma IL-6. J Appl Physiol 95(1): 145–148. 2003.

Horton, TJ, Pagliassotti, MJ, Hobbs, K and Hill, JO. Fuel metabolism in men and women during and after long-duration exercise. J Appl Physiol 85: 1823–1832. 1998.

Huang, D, Ou, B, Hampsch-Woodill, M, Flanagan, JA and Deemer, EK. Development and validation of oxygen radical absorbance capacity assay for lipophilic antioxidants using randomly methylated beta-cyclodextrin as the solubility enhancer. J Agric Food Chem 50(7): 1815–1821. 2002.

Levine, JA, Schleusner, SJ and Jensen, MD. Energy expenditure of nonexercise activity. Am J Clin Nutr 72(6): 1451–1454. 2000.

Ivy, JL, Lee, MC, Broznick, JT and Reed, MJ. Muscle glycogen storage after different amounts of carbohydrate ingestion. J Appl Physiol 65: 2018–2023. 1988.

Jeukendrup, AE and Jentjens, R. Oxidation of carbohydrate feedings during prolonged exercise: Current thoughts, guidelines and directions for future research. Sports Med 29(6): 407–424. 2000.

Jeukendrup, AE, Saris, WH and Wagenmakers, AJ. Fat metabolism during exercise: A review—part III: Effects of nutritional interventions. Int J Sports Med 19(6): 371–379. 1998.

Kerksick, C and Willoughby, D. The antioxidant role of glutathione and N-acetylcysteine supplements and exercise-induced oxidative stress. J Int Soc Sports Nutr 2: 38–44. 2005.

Kovacs, EMR, Stegen, JHCH and Brouns, F. Effect of caffeinated drinks on substrate metabolism, caffeine excretion, and performance. J Appl Physiol 85: 709–715. 1998.

Kreider, RB. Physiological considerations of ultraendurance performance. Int J Sport Nutr 1: 3–27. 1991.

Laursen, PB and Rhodes, EC. Physiological analysis of a high-intensity ultraendurance event. J Strength Conditioning 21: 26–38. 1999.

Laursen, PB and Rhodes, EC. Factors effecting performance in an ultra-endurance triathlon. Sports Med 31: 679–689. 2000.

Law, YL, Ong, WS, GillianYap, TL, Lim, SC and Von Chia, E. Effects of two and five days of creatine loading on muscular strength and anaerobic power in trained athletes. J Strength Cond Res 23(3): 906–914. 2009.

Lehmann, M, et al. Serum amino acid concentrations in nine athletes before and after the 1993 Comar Ultra Triathlon. Int J Sports Med 16(3): 155–159. 1995.

Lindeman, AK. Nutrient intake of an ultraendurance cyclist. Int J Sport Nutr 1: 79–85. 1991.

Lopez, RM, Casa, DJ, McDermott, BP, Ganio, MS, Armstrong, LE and Maresh, CM. Does creatine supplementation hinder exercise heat tolerance or hydration status? A systematic review with meta-analyses. J Athl Train 44(2): 215–223. 2009.

Lopez-Garcia, E, et al. Consumption of (n-3) fatty acids is related to plasma biomarkers of inflammation and endothelial activation in women. J Nutr 134: 1806–1811. 2004.

Machefer, G, et al. Extreme running competition decreases blood antioxidant defense capacity. J Am Coll Nutr 23(4): 358–364. 2004.

Machefer, G, et al. Nutritional and plasmatic antioxidant vitamins status of ultra endurance athletes. J Am Coll Nutr 26(4): 311–316. 2007.

Mackinnon, LT. Chronic exercise training effects on immune function. Med Sci Sports Exerc 32(7 Suppl): S369–376. 2000.

Malczewska, J, Raczynski, G and Stupnicki, R. Iron status in female endurance athletes and in non-athletes. Int J Sport Nutr Exerc Metab 10(3): 260–276. 2000.

Matsumoto, K, Mizuno, M, Mizuno, T, Dilling-Hansen, B, Lahoz, A, Bertelsen, V, Munster, H, Jordening, H, Hamada, K and Doi, T. Branched-chain amino acids and arginine supplementation attenuates skeletal muscle proteolysis induced by moderate exercise in young individual. Int J Sports Med 28: 531–538. 2007.

Maughan, R and Shirreffs, SM. Development of individual hydration strategies for athletes. Int J Sport Nutr Exerc Metab 18: 457–472. 2008

McArdle, WD, Katch, FI and Katch, VL. *Exercise physiology, energy, nutrition, and human performance.* Philadelphia, PA: Lea & Febiger. 1986.

McNaughton, Siegler, J and Midgley, A. Ergogenic effects of sodium bicarbonate. Curr Sports Med Re 7(4): 230–236. 2008.

Melby, CL, Commerford, SR and Hill, JO. Exercise, macronutrient balance, and weight control. In: Lamb DR, Murray R, eds. *Perspectives in exercise science and sports medicine, Vol. 11: Exercise, nutrition and weight control.* Carmel, IN: Cooper Publishing. 1–60. 1998.

Millard-Stafford, ML, Cureston, KJ, Wingo, JE, Trilk, J, Warren, GL and Buyckx, M. Hydration during warm, humid conditions: Effect of a caffeinated sports drink. Int J Sport Nutr Exerc Metab 17(2): 163–177. 2007.

Morillas-Ruiz, J, Zafrilla, P, Almar, M, Cuevas, MJ, Lopez, FJ, Abellan, P, Villegas, JA and Gonzalez-Gallego, J. The effects of an antioxidant-supplemented beverage on exercise-induced oxidative stress: Results from a placebo-controlled double-blind study in cyclists. Eur J Appl Physiol 95(5–6): 543–549. 2005.

Mozaffarian, D, et al. Dietary intake of trans fatty acids and systemic inflammation in women. Am J Clin Nutr 79: 606–612. 2004.

National Athletic Trainers' Association Position Statement: Fluid replacement for athletes. J Athl Train 35: 212–214. 2000.

Nim Han, S, et al. Effect of hydrogenated and saturated, relative to polyunsaturated, fat on immune and inflammatory responses of adults with hypercholesterolemia. J Lipid Res 43: 445–452. 2002.

Nosaka, N, Suzuki, Y, Nagatoishi, A, Kasai, M, Wu, J and Taguchi, M. Effect of ingestion of medium-chain triacylglycerols on moderate- and high-intensity exercise in recreational athletes. J Nutr Sci Vitaminol 55(2): 120–125. 2009.

Ohtani, M, Sugita, M and Maryuma, K. Amino acid mixture improves training efficiency in athletes. J Nutr 136: 538S–543S. 2006.

Ostrowski, K, et al. Pro- and anti-inflammatory cytokine balance in strenuous exercise in humans. J Physiol 515: 287–291. 1999.

Packer, L, Witt, EH and Tritschler, HJ. Alpha-lipoic acid as a biological antioxidant. Free Radic Biol Med 19: 227–250. 1995.

Pai, JK, et al. Inflammatory markers and the risk of coronary heart disease in men and women. N Engl J Med 351: 2599–2610. 2004.

Peake, JM. Vitamin C: Effects of exercise and requirements with training. Int J Sport Nutr Exerc Metab 13: 125–151. 2003.

Peake, JM, Suzuki, K and Coombes, JS. The influence of antioxidant supplementation on markers of inflammation and the relationship to oxidative stress after exercise. J Nutr Biochem 18: 357–371. 2007.

Piehl Aulin, K, Soderlund, K and Hultman, E. Muscle glycogen resynthesis rate in humans after supplementation of drinks containing carbohydrates with low and high molecular masses. Eur J Appl Physiol 81: 346–351. 2000.

Rodenberg, RE and Gustafson, S. Iron as an ergogenic aid: Ironclad evidence? Curr Sports Med Rep 6(4): 258–264. 2007.

Roti, MW, Casa, DJ, Pumerantz, AC, Watson, G, Judelson, DA, Dias, JC, Ruffin, K and Armstrong, LE. Thermoregulatory responses to exercise in the heat: Chronic caffeine intake has no effect. Aviat Space Environ Med 77(2): 124–129. 2006.

Rowlands, DS and Thomson, JS. Effects of beta-hydroxy-beta-methylbutyrate supplementation during resistance training on strength, body composition, and muscle damage in trained and untrained young men: A meta-analysis. J Strength Cond Res 23(3): 836–846. 2009.

Saris, WHM, et al. Study of food intake and energy expenditure during extreme sustained exercise: The Tour de France. Int J Sport Med 10(Suppl): 26–31. 1989.

Sawka, MN, Burke, LM, Eichner, ER, Maughan, RJ, Montain, SJ and Stachenfeld, NS. Exercise and fluid replacement position stand. Med Sci Sports Exerc: 377–389. 2007.

Schaefer, A, Piquard, F, Geny, B, Doutreleau, S, Lampert, E, Mettauer, B and Lonsdorfer, J. L-arginine reduces exercise-induced increase in plasma lactate and ammonia. Int J Sports Med 23: 403–407. 2002.

Sen, CK. Antioxidants in exercise nutrition. Sports Med 31(13): 891–908. 2001.

Shephard, RJ and Shek, PN. Heavy exercise, nutrition and immune function: Is there a connection? Int J Sports Med 8: 491–497. 1995.

Sidossis, LS, Gastaldelli, A, Klein, S and Wolfe, RR. Regulation of plasma fatty acid oxidation during low- and high-intensity exercise. Am J Physiol 272: E1065–1070. 1997.

Speedy, DB, Noakes, TD and Schneider, C. Exercise-associated hyponatremia: A review. Emerg Med 13: 17–27. 2001.

Speich, M, Pineau, A and Ballereau, F. Minerals, trace elements and related biological variables in athletes and during physical activity. Clin Chim Acta 312(1–2): 1–11. 2001.

Stout, JR, et al. Effects of beta- alanine supplementation on the onset of neuromuscular fatigue and ventilatory threshold in women. Amino Acids 32: 381–386. 2007.

Suedekum, NA and Dimeff, RJ. Iron and the athlete. Curr Sports Med Rep 4(4): 199–202. 2005.

Suzuki, Y, Ito, O, Mukai, N and Takahashi, H. High levels of skeletal muscle carnosine contributes to the latter half of exercise performance during 30s maximal cycle ergometer sprinting. Jpn J Physiol 52: 199–205. 2002.

Takanami, Y, Iwane, H, Kawai, Y and Shimomitsu, T. Vitamin E supplementation and endurance exercise: Are there benefits? Sports Med 29(2): 73–83. 2000.

Tarnopolsky, MA, Bosman, M, Macdonald, JR, Vandeputte, D, Martin, J and Roy, BD. Postexercise protein-carbohydrate supplements increase muscle glycogen in men and women. J Appl Physiol 83: 1877–1883. 1997.

Thomson, JS, Watson, PE and Rowlands, DS. Effects of nine weeks of beta-hydroxy-beta-methylbutyrate supplementation on strength and body composition in resistance trained men. J Strength Cond Res 23(3): 827–835. 2009.

Tipton, KD and Wolfe, RR. Protein and amino acids for athletes. J Sports Sci 22: 65–79. 2004.

Turinsky, J and Long, CL. Free amino acids in muscle: Effect of muscle fiber population and denervation. Am J Physiol 258: E485–E491. 1990.

Urso, ML and Clarkson, PM. Oxidative stress, exercise, and antioxidant supplementation. Toxicology 189(1–2): 41–54. 2003.

Vist, GE and Maughan, RJ. Gastric emptying of ingested solutions in man: Effect of beverage glucose concentration. Med Sci Sports Exerc 10: 1269–1273. 1994.

Walberg-Rankin, J. Changing body weights and composition in athletes. In: Lamb, DR, Murray R, eds. *Perspectives in exercise science and sports medicine, Vol. 11: Exercise, nutrition and weight control.* Carmel, IN: Cooper Publishing. 199–236. 1998.

Watson, TA, et al. Antioxidant restriction and oxidative stress in short-duration exhaustive exercise. Med Sci Sports Exerc 37(1): 63–71. 2005.

Wismann J and Willoughby, D. Gender differences in carbohydrate metabolism and carbohydrate loading. J Int Soc Sports Nutr 3: 28–34. 2006.

Woolf, K, Bidwell, WK and Carlson, AG. The effect of caffeine as an ergogenic aid in anaerobic exercise. Int J Sport Nutr Exerc Metab 18(4): 412–429. 2008.

Woolf, K, Bidwell, WK and Carlson, AG. Effect of caffeine as an ergogenic aid during anaerobic exercise performance in caffeine naïve collegiate football players. J Strength Cond Res 23(5): 1363–1369. 2009.

Yeo, SE, Jentjens, RL, Wallis, GA and Jeukendrup, AE. Caffeine increases exogenous carbohydrate oxidation during exercise. J Appl Physiol 99(3): 844–850. 2005.

Zoeller, RF, Stout, JR, O'Kroy, JA, Torok, DJ and Mielke, M. Effects of 28 days of beta-alanine and creatine monohydrate supplementation on aerobic power, ventilatory and lactate thresholds, and time to exhaustion. Amino Acids 33: 505–510. 2006.

Index

Note: *Italic* page numbers indicate illustrations, text boxes, and tables or charts.

About the Author

Bob Seebohar, MS, RD, CSSD, CSCS

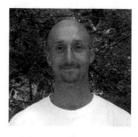

Bob Seebohar has worn many hats throughout his career. Starting out as an exercise physiologist by studying exercise and sports science in his undergraduate work, he turned to the fitness world upon exiting college. However, he soon found himself asking more questions than he could answer, so he decided to return to graduate school to expand his knowledge base. He received his first graduate degree in health and exercise science with an emphasis on metabolism; it was during this time that he was formally introduced to sports nutrition. Throughout graduate school, Bob worked with collegiate athletes, assisting them in improving their health and performance through nutrition, and it was then that he realized that he had discovered his true passion of combining exercise with nutrition.

This led Bob to staying in graduate school another year to receive a second graduate degree in food science and human nutrition, mostly to satisfy the qualifications of becoming a Registered Dietitian (RD). He knew that he would require that expertise to continue his work with athletes. After graduate school, Bob was extremely focused on becoming one of the best sport dietitians in the country and outlined a specific plan to attain this goal. Throughout the past 16 years, he has acquired valuable hands-on experience, working with athletes of all ages and abilities, and has fine-tuned his approach to sports nutrition. He has worked in the collegiate sports nutrition setting as a consultant to Colorado State University and the University of Northern Colorado, has held the position of Director of Sports Nutrition at the University of Florida, and was a sport dietitian for the U.S. Olympic Committee, where he was fortunate to travel to the 2008 Olympics as a sport dietitian.

Bob is known to think outside the box and politely challenge the "why's" behind the way things work. These two traits have brought Bob's work to the attention of many high-caliber athletes and coaches and fellow health professionals. He is considered to be a thought-provoking sport dietitian who constantly strives for excellence in his work with athletes by always attempting to leave no stone unturned when it comes to improving performance. Currently, Bob provides sports nutrition services to all types of athletes—including endurance, strength, power, and aesthetic/skills—through his company, Fuel4mance (www.fuel4mance.com).

In addition to his sport nutrition emphasis, Bob is one of the foremost experts on strength training for endurance athletes and holds the NSCA Certified Strength and Conditioning Specialist certification. He is also a USA Triathlon Level III Elite Coach, having worked with Susan Williams, 2004 Olympic Triathlon Bronze Medalist, as her strength coach and sport dietitian; as coach and sport dietitian to Sarah Haskins, 2008 Olympian in triathlon; and coach and sport dietitian of Jasmine Oeinck, 2009 Elite National Champion triathlete.

Practicing what he preaches, Bob is a competitive athlete himself. Growing up playing soccer for 18 years, he shifted his focus (on a dare) to endurance competitions in 1993 and has not looked back since. He has competed in hundreds of multi-sport races, most notably six Ironman races, the Boston Marathon, the Leadville 100-mile mountain bike race, and the Leadville 100-mile trail run. In 2009, he became a Leadman, completing a series of ultra-endurance events that included a marathon, 50-mile mountain bike race, 50-mile trail run, 100-mile mountain bike race, 10-kilometer run, and 100-mile run, all in a span of 7 weeks at altitudes of 10,200 feet and above. The longer and more challenging the endeavor, the better. Bob truly believes in taking his body to its physical, mental, and nutritional boundaries. He is truly a "walk the talk" sport dietitian and has a keen understanding of the physical, mental, and nutritional components that it takes to be a successful athlete.